CW01502032

SEXUAL CYSTITIS

Angela Kilmartin was born in Essex. On leaving school she worked as a fashion model for some years and then studied at the Guildhall School of Music and Drama on singing and acting scholarships. In 1966 she married, and started disabling attacks of cystitis, complicated by thrush caused by continuous antibiotics. Five years later cystitis had put an end to her promising singing career and created tremendous difficulties in her marriage.

Then one urologist introduced her to self-help and a dramatic return to health. Angered by the lack of this simple advice over her five years of cystitis, Angela founded the famous U and I Club in 1971, a registered charity for teaching prevention and management of urinary problems to both patients and doctors. By 1980 both her books were available **worldwide** and the U and I Club was stopped.

The acknowledged authority on self-help in cystitis, she has, among other efforts, toured the USA for television and radio shows, lectured worldwide, made films, instigated the Health Education Council leaflet on cystitis, and has now written five bestselling books on cystitis.

Angela has now returned to live in London after following her husband on postings to Nigeria and Saudi Arabia. She lectures and counsels on cystitis and enjoys solo oratorio work with choral societies around the country.

SEXUAL
CYSTITIS

Angela Kilmartin

ARROW BOOKS

*This book is for my son, Rory, in the hope
that he will, as a knowing man, lovingly
share with his wife the joys of healthy sex.*

Arrow Books Limited
62–65 Chandos Place, London WC2N 4NW

An imprint of Century Hutchinson Limited

London Melbourne Sydney Auckland
Johannesburg and agencies throughout the world

First published in 1988

© Angela Kilmartin 1988
Illustrations by Pat Ludlow and Tony Morris

Printed and bound in Great Britain by
The Guernsey Press Co. Ltd., Guernsey, Channel Islands.

ISBN 0 09 955690 1

Contents

Part II: Having Intercourse

Part III: After Intercourse

Acknowledgements

My thanks are due to The Spinal Injuries Association and The Rape Crisis Centre.

Also to Mr Desmond Bluett, FRCS, FRCOG, for his unfailing support and superb skills; to Mr and Mrs Peter Wright and Miss Jenny Nicholls for their frank talking; Miss Jane Usher for the emergency typing and to my children for all their comments!

AK

Forethought

If you've just picked up this book on a shelf and think that cystitis is only caused by sex, you couldn't be more wrong. This is just one aspect of cystitis so look along the shelf for my other books if necessary.

Cystitis, as I'm given to saying on every possible occasion, is just a symptom of something else wrong. Find the something else wrong and you stand an excellent chance of stopping the cystitis.

Many more women than men get cystitis and four out of five women will experience it at some stage in their lives. It can start literally at any time from birth to death for an infinite number of reasons but there are some points in the female's cycle when she would appear to be more at risk.

These points are:

1 Childhood.
2 Puberty.
3 Onset of regular sexual relations.
4 Pregnancy.
5 Childbirth.
6 Menopause.
7 Hysterectomy.
8 Old Age.

In this book I propose to look in great detail at point three, sexual cystitis, although, having mentioned seven others, it might be helpful to explain them a little more. Until you get your first-ever attack, there is no reason whatsoever to search for or take note of anything written on the subject. Indeed many women, especially young ones, don't even know the condition exists until they experience it first-hand. Then they panic because of embarrassment and, later through fear of it happening again.

The symptoms of cystitis are, classically:

1 Pain on passing urine.
2 Frequency of passing urine.
3 Bleeding from the urethra whilst passing urine.
4 Fever.
5 Back ache.
6 Nausea.

Not everyone experiences all these symptoms. You can have only two or three of them, in any order or any severity from just nuisance value through to mind-blowing agony. Young sufferers go to the doctor fast but older ones will learn to use a combination of self-help and medical help. Over the past twenty years, countless magazines and newspaper articles, television and radio programmes have promoted my ideas on prevention and management of urinary problems. Leaflets and lectures now push hospitals and health-centre doctors into extolling the values and virtues of managing cystitis in a preventative fashion rather than by senseless operations and needless antibiotics.

I consider that eighty per cent of attacks of cystitis or similar urinary conditions are self-caused quite unwittingly by the patient. It therefore follows that eighty per cent of attacks of cystitis or similar urinary conditions can be stopped or at least controlled by the patient when someone has given her the wits to do so.

The remaining twenty per cent of cases do require medical help *but* such help has to be very carefully administered in a tailor-made way to meet an individual's need and is usually of a gynaecological nature. Urological investigations prove invariably negative.

Just because your cystoscopy (bladder and urethral examination under anaesthetic) shows inflammation, don't run away thinking that this in itself is an illness or an answer. It only means that something is upsetting the linings – you have yet to discover what that 'something' is!

IVPs (intravenous pyelogram – X-ray) of the kidneys, bladder and urethra are also usually negative for most women with cystitis. In fifteen years of counselling, I have yet to meet a patient with positive kidney X-rays showing stones or deformities or cancer. This is because anything like this will have been dealt with immediately by the urologist who requested the X-ray and no such women ever find their way to me. Such urological problems, even at medical level, are the exception rather than a rule and such patients of the female gender are few and far between.

MSUs (mid-stream urine samples) are of the utmost importance and *must* be taken for proper analysis. Whatever the result, it is vital to know it and it is the first major clue for any line of investigation. Bacterial causes of cystitis are entirely preventable and so are large numbers of non-bacterial causes, but unless you *know* what is in your own urine sample you can't begin to work on the routines or suggestions in this book or any of my others.

Vaginal swabs and cervical swabs are *always* a good idea. Insist on having them and on knowing the result. FPA doctors and VD specialists sadly only look for their speciality diseases or conditions, and too many doctors don't bother about discharges from cervical erosions or polyps. Gynaecological interest in mundane vaginal health is at an all-time low and patients deserve better treatment in this area.

It is a good rule to be suspicious of medical terminology – the 'urethral syndrome' is just one such, or 'non-specific urethitis'. Both simplified mean 'nothing specific' and 'undefined': in other words 'we don't know'.

It's also a good rule to steer absolutely clear of urological operations like urethral dilations unless at least one other urologist agrees with the first one and they both have the same foolproof medical reason for wanting to stretch your urethra and bladder. Dilations scar the linings of the bladder and urethra and muscle strength is lost on the scar. The failure rate of dilations to improve cystitis is enormous. This operation is mostly only performed as a fob off. Beware!

There is just no medical excuse for operating on a cystitis patient when one kidney X-ray and one cystoscopy have both come up negative. Common sense is all!

It is far better to ask a straightforward question: When did your cystitis start?

If it started, say, when you were seventeen years old, it's safe to assume that your bladder worked perfectly well up to then, therefore nothing of a serious nature can be causing the cystitis. This assumption would be backed up by a negative X-ray and negative cystoscopy.

In fact, if your bladder has worked perfectly well up to *any* age and your kidney X-ray and cystoscopy are negative, you can still assume there is nothing seriously wrong and that the attacks will be redeemable with the appropriate specialist help.

Redeeming such attacks – stopping them – lies first and foremost, as I said, in finding the cause of them. To have nothing that is medically serious is often a great frustration to victims of cystitis. They long to be diagnosed and for the doctor to find something wrong in order that he can put it right. The doctor gets very frustrated about it, too, and until self-help and prevention came along with my work, patients were given heavy and extended doses of antibiotics with dreadful side effects. Long term courses of tranquillizers and many unnecessary dilations had no effect either. The cystitis still wouldn't stop!

Frankly, there's no excuse these days to get frustrated. If you have picked up this book you'll know that the author understands how you feel, and if you don't think your cystitis is sexually related then get one of my other books. You really aren't alone: millions of women the world over get cystitis and know just what you're going through. Frustration comes from lack of knowledge. There's plenty of knowledge available these days if you look on the bookshelves.

So you've found my book and you're going to learn – next problem: your doctor! I'd like a pound for every time I've heard a woman say 'My doctor is so unhelpful.' Is he though?

Has he tested your urine?   Yes.
Has he sent you for a kidney X-ray?   Yes.
Has he sent you to a urologist?   Yes.
Has he given you a leaflet on cystitis?   Yes/No.
Has he prescribed antibiotics?   Yes.

Well that's all quite normal, useful and helpful. He's doing the basics of a good job.

Has he sent you to a gynaecologist?   No.
Has he given you the title of a good book to read on the subject?   No.
Has he told you what's in your urine sample?   No.
Has he told you to start helping yourself?   No.

Well that's not so helpful.

Have *you* asked specifically for your urine results?   No.
Have *you* asked if he has a leaflet?   No.
Have *you* asked for the title of a good book on
  cystitis?   No.

Why not? All doctors these days recognize the value of
such groups as Alcoholics Anonymous, the Mastectomy
Association, the Migraine Trust, the Asthma Council and
so on. Why stop at the bladder? The old U & I Club, a
charity for cystitis sufferers and closed in 1981, has been
replaced by my books, lectures and counselling. The self-
help is still here and growing enormously, and a support
group is unnecessary and unwise in this case. Why
shouldn't your GP recognize the value of your co-operation on your own cystitis?
Having found a good book –
Have you shown it to your GP?   No.

So mightn't your GP be pleased to see your efforts to help
yourself, and also to assist him? Getting you better isn't
solely your GP's job – it's also yours. Take more responsibility for your health and remove some of your GP's
workload. It's a different viewpoint, isn't it? Suddenly
there's an alternative to sitting in the waiting room. Maybe
it's you who's not being helpful. Had you thought of that?
  Medical education is a continuous process. In every
surgery, every day, a good doctor will still be learning.
He learns from medical magazines, patient's reports,
laboratory reports and drug company representatives. He
attends courses, reads medical papers and reads books.
In the last fifteen years great numbers of books have been
written by patients or doctors with particularly vested
interests, and there is a tremendous toing and froing of
information. Cystitis is one of the commonest female
complaints and your GP will be very thankful to have new
information on it. Plonk one of my books on his desk.

During my eight years of living overseas in Lagos and Jeddah, one of the great sustaining influences of such difficult places was 'ladies' lunches'. These sometimes simple, sometimes formal – but always good for a laugh – events, were a major factor in communicating and relaying information. A good gossip is informative and instructive – and it can also be exhausting as we laughed so much. They say that laughter is a tonic, and I have every reason to verify that. Those women supported each other sometimes knowingly, but often unknowingly, just by their companionship and laughter.

I have now been back in the UK for four years and my 'ladies' lunches' are no longer regular events, but two or three times a year I say, 'To hell with it all I'm having a ladies lunch!' Nothing in my life at this time is more fun than a few women released from the daily cares of professional or domestic duties and gossiping over a good meal at home.

On my birthday I phoned five friends of my own age, two of whom I have known from school, and all six of us settled down to a good update and gossip. Feeling the atmosphere about right, midway through the main course and the second glass of wine, I hesitantly asked them if they thought they were sufficiently knowledgeable about sex when they got married.

If they had been under a conductor's baton they couldn't have made a better combined entry: *No!* And, 'I didn't know anything you say, Angela, in your books.'

'Didn't your mother tell you anything?'

'*No!*'

'How many of you washed before or after sex?'

Two out of the five had washed – one without thinking about it, and one because she had done some nursing. And so it went on, but not, unfortunately, long enough to do a real in-depth survey. The phone interrupted, the

15

potatoes needed passing, the latest baby dropped his spoon etc.

I asked a neighbour if she had known to wash before or after sex and she said that she had only known to wash afterwards. She knew because she'd worked in a local bank and all the women brought rolls and coffee for lunch and sat in a group. Intimate information was often exchanged and from this group my neighbour had learned a few things about sex.

I never learned anything about sex before I courted. My mother had done her duty over menstruation, but the relationship between us was not close enough to accommodate sexual discussions. At school in the 'fifties we learned about the reproductive system of the rabbit and it never entered our heads to contemplate male/female human reproduction, let alone sexuality. I had no brothers or sisters, so was disadvantaged in this area also. Not for me listening at the door to older discussions!

Magazines in the 'sixties never mentioned cystitis or sexual matters and *Lady Chatterley's Lover*, lent to me one weekend by an older model girl from one of the fashion-houses where I worked, was a positive mental disturbance! The first penis ever to be brought into my view caused nausea, weak knees and the fast exit of one amazed and disappointed lad from the kitchen. I was a 'good girl'.

I was also a very ignorant girl! I didn't like to ask anyone about anything and there was nothing to read. It was the same story for many girls in those days.

For the past fifteen years or so, there have been attempts in schools all over the world to give a recognisable sex education. It's a very variable education and can be dependant upon the willingness or the capability of any one teacher, the nearness of a trained sex educator or counsellor and, most of all, the agreement of the head, the school staff, the parents and maybe even the governors to allow it within the curriculum.

The content of the lessons will take into account such considerations as whether it's a single-sex school or coeducational; the best age group to start the children; whether to hold the lessons in small groups or take the whole class together and, according to all this, then precisely what sort of things to say to them.

Once started, of course, children from thirteen years upwards want to know everything, often because they have older brothers or sisters and in some cases because the girls have already been persuaded to start intercourse. There are magazines and comics, aimed at a teenage readership, which can be bought with pocket money on any bookstall, and whose articles encourage the hero-worship of pop personalities. Suggestive songs and dancing in figure-hugging clothes – these all lead to the heightening of sexual excitement and arousal in the young. Soap operas, plays, movies, medical programmes and advertisements all add to the hyping up of the young to become far more interested in sex than we have seen in many generations.

Contraceptives, whilst still regarded with horrifying casualness by young people today, are, nevertheless, there for use. Condoms, vaginal sponges, spermicidal jellies, creams and foams can be bought over the counter and even regular sexual activity can be catered for by going on the Pill at an early age.

Homosexuality has become open. The more open it has become, the more such knowledge has reached teenagers who would otherwise never have heard of it, let alone indulged in it. In many inner-city schools around the world, teachers have openly expressed their ideas and brought the subject under the umbrella of sex education. Children's minds have never been so besieged by sexual ideas and manners. The media, magazines and teachers have in the name of progress assaulted our children's minds and hearts in hitherto unpractised ways. The way teachers behave both in and out of the classroom is as important as the behaviour of parents and family members. Such adults are in contact with children during all the formative years, when a child's mind is at its most receptive.

Many inner-city teachers and inner-city parents tend to create inner-city offspring – streetwise and sexually strident. Modern travel and racial integration has led to a confusion and babel of social and sexual interchange.

Imported drugs encourage and stimulate the shyest of strangers to indulge in sexual activities, and late-night porn movies in hotels or on videos at home stimulate dark corners of the mind to 'try it out'.

Time was when the sailor ashore in an exotic port would wander the back alleys, indulge himself and return to wife and family months later, all memories of the indulgence committed to his memory bank and his alone. Last year, thanks to television and the curiousity of the camera, we, the great public, went ashore with him and were transported into a world of easy-sell sex where for a dime a young Far Eastern sex girl serving liquor took out from her leopardskin T-shirt the breast of the sailor's choice and we all saw him take two or three long sucks on the nipple while she held it. There was much giggling, laughter and ribaldry from his mates who queued for their turn. She then tucked the breast away and served another drink!

Such scenes in a prime-time travelogue of a luxury cruise ship happened with sneaky quickness – not time enough to turn the fourteen-year-old out of the room. So millions of people in their own homes watching a travel programme were given an exotic piece of sex education. This year I've lost count of the numbers of films and plays where cameras carefully sited in semi-darkened rooms have witnessed glistening white male buttocks rising to an assortment of rhythms in simulation – I presume simulation – of penetration and orgasm. Its the in-thing now and I suppose makes a change from the gleaming clenched teeth, knitted eyebrows and ecstatic hands of the woman underneath kneading his shoulders!

All of this is sex education, make no mistake about it. Sex education is certainly no longer a confined curricular or parental subject to be brought up over the dishwashing or at eleven o'clock on Tuesday morning after history! The media is very heavily involved.

No wonder that parents in the past thirty years or so have opted out of telling their children the facts of sex. In these particular years sex became a magazine subject, a media subject and parents felt their own contribution to be off the mark, probably irrelevant, or not nearly so interestingly presented. Feature writers or book authors were welcome to take their place and do their job for them! Teachers of the new-wave 'sixties and 'seventies' progressive schools started the school sex education programmes, and parents again largely stood by and opted out.

Dr Henry Ritter, an American MD, writing in his book *From Man to Man* says, 'Parents have an obligation *to learn* how to play their roles as the primary sex educators.'

That is a very telling sentence. Parental obligation is extensive. It isn't enough to feed, clothe, love and house your children. You must set standards, give guidance, lay down right and wrong and make sure that your children know about their own bodies and how the human race is procreated. Only word of mouth ever achieved this before the twentieth century, and a few books. Parental intercourse in a shared bedroom might have given some practical instruction to unsleepy eyes and would have been the trigger for a simple direct question 'What was Dad doing to you last night? I wasn't asleep so I saw,' but children usually sleep in another room these days.

You are *obliged by parenthood* to teach your child about sex. You are the best person and you must not let your child down. More than ever in history it is absolutely vital to give clear guidance and instruction on healthy sexual activity. Only you know your individual children and their current state of enquiry or receptivity. It doesn't matter if the nature of wordage of a child's sexual question is funny. They know they sometimes don't express their general questions in an adult way and that the adult smiles or laughs. If you are seen to try to hide a laugh at a sexual query or try to be dismissive and wary, they'll know and feel dissatisfied. They may not trust you again.

Laugh if you must, explain why you've laughed, put your arms around their shoulders for a quick spontaneous hug and then collect yourself ready to give a straight answer to them.

Just such an occasion happened to me and my twelve-year-old son, to whom this book is dedicated. We were motoring back to his prep school on a spring Sunday evening deep in chatter, and there was a pause.

'You know what's going to happen next term?' he asked.

'Cricket', I replied, manoeuvring into the outside lane.

'Apart from that, I mean. We're going to be taught about the dreaded S-E-X.'

'What, sex education?'

'Yup, Mr Cope the science master's going to do it.'

'Oh well,' I said, regaining the inner lane and much interested in what he had just revealed, 'Would it be a good idea to tell you some of the names of the male and female parts of the reproductive organs so that you go with some accurate advance information?'

'Oh no, we all know the names – it's just we've no idea where they all go.'

I roared and roared with laughter as the image of sixteen little boys whispering inaccurate sitings of the testicles and womb sprang into mind!

Assured by my temporary leave of senses, he proudly

boasted that he knew there were four hundred different words for penis and how many did I know?

'Certainly not that many.'

Much emboldened, he began on some that he knew and we started a two-way exchange of information. I took over then, and some twenty minutes later had him not only in full command of the geography of both male and female reproductive organs, but also how part of one set went into part of the other set, what each part was used for and how the words were spelt.

As we pulled off the motorway, he had the lot off absolutely pat right through to Fallopian tubes! I ended with the guarded advice to confine his knowledge to the S-E-X class and that really sex talk was best done within a confidential atmosphere. Not during assembly, for instance, just as talk of cricket or baseball in a music appreciation class is out of place. In other words, there's a time and a place for everything in life.

I'm not of the view that adults parade nakedness in their home, I don't except in my bedroom when dressing. If one of the children walks in for some reason there's usually a cry of 'What a sight!'

The 'sight' continues unabashed to search for bra and pants in some tangled drawer and replies along the lines of 'Don't mock the afflicted.' . . . 'It's all I've got' . . . 'What can I do for you?' . . . 'If you can't stand it don't stay!'

There's no embarrassment, but equally there's no unnecessary flaunting on the landings or elsewhere. Bathrooms are understood in our home to be places where people generally prefer to be alone, but if instructions have to be given, for instance, regarding emergency supplies from the corner shop then it's quite all right to come in if permission is given by the bather.

At fourteen my daughter firmly locked the bathroom door and it remains so. She will hesitantly turn her back whilst trying on a newly bought dress even though she's now nineteen. No-one laughs or tries to tell her she's prudish – she is respected for her own wishes. For many years she has heard much about the male and female body because of my work, and has lived with expressions like 'urine', 'faecal material', 'vaginal bruising' and so on. She has come with me into studios for TV programmes and she has read about my work both in my own books and other people's features on it. She has once watched me on stage at a medical lecture discussing cystitis and we have always had a quite open line on sex talk, but before she started university we had a final intimate conversation about the act of intercourse itself and the way in which sexual organs should be cared for. In view of all my experiences, I must know that she is as well prepared for sex as I can possibly make her. I want for my daughter what I myself have not had through my own ignorance and illness and my husband's absences: a happy, healthy, regular sex life.

My sex life didn't begin until late courtship and engagement. It was not orgasmic or fulfilling – no early sex is. From the third day of my honeymoon I was out of sexual action because of cystitis. The next five years of intense attacks every three to four weeks and lasting two to three weeks meant an all-consuming existence of pain, incontinence, operations, antibiotics, vaginal thrush, examinations, three periods of six months each without sex, on doctor's orders. There was terrible fear, too. Fear of the next attack and the ensuing sexual deprivation, the rows, the distress and, of course, the physical symptoms to which one never became accustomed. They were just as terrible each time. Don't be fooled by anyone who proclaims cystitis is an inconvenience. This problem can devastate a perfectly good marriage and wreck a career. After those five years, my vaginal health was also in tatters with regular trouble. To make matters worse my husband developed severe lip herpes and we barely kissed for three years, never mind had regular weekly sex. Then in 1975, after nine years of sexual disaster, he went with his company to Lagos for three years. We met intermittently and in those three years I only lived in Lagos for eighteen months. The company provided twin beds and my husband refused to approach his managing director for a double bed for fear of putting himself forward, so I spent those eighteen months in a twin bed.

After Lagos we went to Jeddah and, with a lot of other marital trouble vastly exacerbated by memories of twin beds, money troubles and sparse sex, the marriage fell badly apart with sex occurring only once or twice every two to four months, if that. For two years prior to the divorce, sex between us was non-existent.

So for these briefly explained reasons, with much left out, I am determined to give my daughter an enlightened chance of greater sexual happiness. If, in so doing, I write this latest book with the future sexual wellbeing of my daughter and son in mind, then I am writing for the best – and what is good enough for both of them may also be good enough for you, the reader, and your family and friends.

It is still news for a sex book to be written by a woman. Slowly we are putting on paper our ideas, and not necessarily looking to male writers to 'tell us all'. I hope that this book will discuss the real intimacies of sexual health, not just state the technicalities and geographies.

Sexual bonding in early marriage is something seldom mentioned, but perhaps it can be likened to good cement between the assorted bricks of life. If the cement is absent or of poor quality, the bricks can be blown over. Equally, too much cement and not enough bricks can end with a large boring lump of concrete much like a tower block and liable to structural collapse.

If you go to the trouble of marrying these days, or even

of commencing a conscientious live-in, then take time out to sexually bond together. Don't put the office first and leave half an hour at midnight for a swift hump! You and your partner deserve better. Good sex takes thought, energy, weekends off and lots of love. Frequent casual sex sets fake standards, yardsticks and expectations. It can make bonding with someone really special very much harder later on, and make the habit of sleeping around difficult to break or refuse.

Men, mostly, have always slept casually. Women also now participate in far greater numbers. The 'nice girls' now do it and enjoy it and, like the men, are finding that it is hard, once married, to stop the old habits. Mary Whitehouse, a brave woman, said, 'Adultery *can't* be a good thing because it never ends happily.' She's right, and all of us know that in our hearts. She didn't say it first though – it was written down on two tablets called the Ten Commandments and handed to Charlton Heston up a fake mountain in the film of that name! And before Charlton Heston, Moses received those commandments in fire from God – so the Bible tells us.

If it was that important that long ago, it probably still is today. The using of contraceptives only stops the baby, it doesn't stop the deceit, loss of trust and great unhappiness.

Sleep casually and you sleep uneasily. Things have gone too far to say categorically to young people, *'Don't* have intercourse before marriage,' but it is nevertheless worthwhile to bear in mind the dangers of ill health, unhappiness, embarrassment and loss of trust in partners who prove to be very experienced lovers! With whom and with how many have they learnt their skills? And are they only currently involved with you or are you just for Tuesdays?

In the Moslem Koran the low incidence of sexual activity between a husband and wife can be cited as grounds for divorce. It says that a wife should be penetrated a

24

minimum of once every six weeks for her health, welfare and the continuation of the marital state. Not to be penetrated within that six weeks can be legal grounds for marital breakdown. Once, on a long-haul to Jeddah, I chanced to sit next to a Catholic woman. We spent five hours chatting and at one point I said that I was pleased to be returning just to have some sex because it was twelve weeks since my husband and I had last been together. This started off quite a few confidences and it emerged that both of us could manage up to six weeks without sex but after that our breasts flattened, we slept less well and were quicker to nag the children. Interesting that the Koran – centuries old – considers six weeks a yardstick as well as two modern western women!

Make no bones about it, *life* will be the determining force in your sex life. Of course, moments will come when you are in charge and have the choice to accept, refuse, or postpone any given person or situation. But over the years, as they progress, you will start to judge by these past experiences whether your sex life is happy. I once filled in a woman's magazine survey on a train journey. It was marked in terms of colours, not numbers. Black was bad, red was ecstatically happily. The best I could answer was pale grey going to moments of black with a lot of dark grey – eighteen years of it.

Only two alterations in my life would have been needed to put my colour marks up into the bright red category:

1 I should have known to pass water after intercourse and not get my brand of sexual cystitis.
2 I should have fought with all my might my ex-husband's decision to work abroad.

Look very much more carefully at sex and health and other decisions. Take advice, ask for it, see a marriage guidance counsellor at times of decisions even in the stable marriage. Avoidance of trouble and the prevention of sexual distress is something that must be learnt very early.

I did take advice on the upbringing of my children *before* I even married. I looked around at the children of friends and asked the mother of those whom I considered to be the best brought up, and the nicest children to be with, whether she had any special words of wisdom to offer on their upbringing and her attitude to them. She had:

> 'If you lose control of them within the first fortnight of their life you're lost forever.'

Very deep words, but I remembered and it has paid off. My children and I are very close and loving, and they have done well at school. They are welcomed everywhere and I feel I can take them everywhere.

It never, sadly, ever once occurred to me to ask advice, real intimate advice, from any happily married couple about sex, love and marriage. Determination of many parents to be seen 'not interfering' has made me equally determined to watch over my children's future marriages; to actively open doors before and during those marriages where they can seek detailed, confidential and intimate help. That help could easily take the form of suggesting they see someone else in a given speciality, not me just giving my own opinions.

As more and more family units break down and increases continue in one-parent families, we see plain unremitting distress as there are fewer trusted people from whom to learn happy ways. Build up the units again, educate and love children, open lines of learning and talking to one another, aim for better and more frequent happy sexual intercourse – all of this and much more can only be beneficial.

Look at the following letter, just look at it! Had I been doing my work on cystitis twenty-eight years ago, I would have changed this woman's life. Her cystitis obviously started when sexual intercourse began, and I know that my teachings would have stopped it.

Dear Angela,

I just thought I would write to you about my twenty-eight years of married life. I read one of your books about three years ago and lent it to a friend but never got it back. I think you could write a book about me as my surgeon has often told me to write one.

I was watching Breakfast Television this morning sitting on a bucket for one and a half hours, as I do most mornings because my toilet is upstairs and I can not get to it in time, when you came on the screen.

I started off with cystitis straight after my marriage. I was at the doctor's every three to four weeks getting tablets. My husband had to take some as well and we were unable to have sex for a week. I had a baby one year after our marriage and then cystitis carried on every three to four weeks and I carried on taking tablets.

I went back to the doctor and he said that I should take the Pill to stop it, but it didn't. I didn't get it quite so often but I still suffered terribly.

I lost my Dad in August this year. The surgeon told me he was going to die with a brain tumour right on his retirement after forty-three years working. That shocked my whole body. My body resisted the tablets as the shock goes to your weak spot and boy did I suffer!

I have been in hospital twenty-five times in the eight years after his death.

Tests, cystitis, biopsies, fourteen catheters, bladder wash-outs where I had to lay on my back for three days and have nitrate pumped into my bladder, where all the stuff used to come out in great big lumps with blood on it like a kettle that got scaled up, up to thirty-six bottles! The pain was unbearable sometimes but it had to be done. I also had a hysterectomy six years ago.

I have had three nervous breakdowns from 1982–83 then 1985–86. I was in hospital from 17 November until 11 February

1986. I have just got over that and I am now waiting to go into hospital again under Mr [Blank] the top surgeon to have my bladder taken out and a plastic one put in. What else he is going to find I do not know as I am in so much pain. I really have suffered. I am told that I am a young looking fifty-year-old.

I have just retired from working at British Home Stores after sixteen years through ill health. I get a bit of a pension which I paid in. My husband has also lost his job at fifty-two years old. My daughter gets married on 7 September and my own marriage has just about ended.

With all the other things I have to do I have to look after my mother who is on tablets and is like a walking zombie, I am nearly going round the bend with worry over the operation. I have just about had enough, as your body can only stand so much. What do you think?

I hope you don't mind me writing to you to tell you about everything, I don't think anyone else could have suffered so much and still look so good. It is a wonder that I am not as grey as a badger.

I can't sit down very well as I am always doing housework, and I go dancing. I can't go swimming, biking, or walk very far as I am always wet through and I have to wear Pampers to stop it coming through my clothes.

I hope for a bed anytime after next week as the surgeon was fully booked up in March and April. When I went to see him, I asked, 'What am I going to do for another eight weeks?' He said' Just keep wearing the padding and weeing'. I said, 'Great, I've been doing that for nine years.'

So there is my story, but there is a lot more to it besides – like riding in a car and weeing in bags and baby pads. Then stopping at garages to throw it away because there are no toilets on motorways. I have always gone behind trees otherwise.

I hope you don't mind me writing to you, but I have always wanted to see you and I did this morning, which I enjoyed very much.

Anyway, Angela, thank you for reading my letter and maybe I will hear from you.

Thank you again.
Mrs S.Y.
South Humberside.

I find the most telling sentence in this awful tale the one that starts in the third paragraph: 'I started off with cystitis straight away after my marriage.' Nothing else should have ever happened to her because her bladder was quite untroublesome before that. Doctors and drugs added to her early troubles.

I've written this book precisely to help Mrs S.Y. and millions of other young women. Do heed what I say: I know, because I'm now old enough to know, that marriages fail and sexual unhappiness occurs for an infinite number of reasons. I can help all women to enjoy better sexual health – well, we're all good at something, I'm good at this!

So read on. Put qualms aside and decide from now on to promote good sexual health, not just for yourself but for any young person or miserable acquaintance as well. I've found I'm a good teacher, so put your trust in my twenty years of knowledge and working experience and let me tell you a thing or two you may not have known about sexual health.

The Vagina Et Al

There is little doubt left in my mind that the vagina was not intended to be so frequently used. We almost *ab*use it today. You don't have to be a university professor to see that contraceptives have changed the role of the vagina for all time. Its purpose for being within the female body was and is to facilitate fertilization of eggs and to be a passage for the birth of a baby from the warm womb to the cold room.

Now look what it has to put up with! The expectation, at least, and the frequent performance of, non-conceptive pleasurable humping!

Everytime that a penis is inserted, surrounding tubes and organs in the female have to find somewhere else to go whilst it takes up space and hammers away in ecstatic frenzy. The penis, being outside the male body at all times, doesn't have to be so accommodating and in the male, there are no other organs in proximity needing to displace themselves.

Several sessions of this activity a week make unacceptable and sometimes impossible demands upon the bodies of many women. All sorts of bodily rebellions and alarm signals go out: tight, swollen breasts that hurt and need a larger bra, tiredness that impedes decision-making and work tolerance, tetchy moods, changes in urinary output, sore skin and cystitis.

Expectation of intercourse is now as much a social habit as a necessity of sexual relief. The young girl, newly adult or newly married, is *expected* to be very sexually active. Her boyfriend *expects* to have a lot of sex – that's what he's got her for, that's why he's given up all his nights with the boys and let her move into his flat or vice versa. Young men can have a prodigious output of erections and orgasms and have no hesitation in finding a freely available vagina, protected against pregnancy. There are so many about these days.

The freely available vagina, protected against pregnancy, is much more willing than it ever was twenty years ago. Good contraception, and ready abortion, if mistakes occur, give every woman the freedom to be willing, if she wants. She does want. Women now *want* almost as much as the men! Suddenly, after all these centuries of human existence, the vagina has found its own sensuality and sensitivity. Holidays, central heating and more money mean more time for relaxing, and there's nothing like a good hump in pleasant circumstances to prove an enjoyable pastime – and one which is repeatable ad infinitum.

Sexy clothes, erotic dancing, word of mouth, magazines, music all tell her she can. She can have intercourse whenever, wherever and with whomsoever it pleases her. Mother no longer says, 'Wait till you're married.' This is a major human biological revolution – early and repeated use of the simple birth canal solely for pleasure. Where will such activity lead?

We know it leads to more cancer of the cervix, but will it in tens of thousands of years' time lead to biological reproductive changes? It took that long and several changes of climate for body hair to be less necessary, and therefore lessen in subsequent generations. Will the over-use of the vagina and the battering of the cervix lead to some lessening of egg output, for instance, with a subsequent dive in the birth rate? It's a fascinating thought.

We are coming close to redundancy of marriage and moral scruples. Cases can be argued all ways for moral scruples, or for complete sexual freedom.

The vagina and cervix, already under pressure, are beginning to show just what sorts of illnesses they can think of to put such freedom out of reach. Look what Aids is doing to homosexual activity. Death after seven years is a lethal outcome of the thoughtless use of a part of the body that was not intended for such use. The anus and lower bowel have one use and one use only: excretion of waste body products and poisons, not penile intercourse.

Nature frequently deals with the over-productive woman. Her reproductive organs become weakened and in poorer areas such a woman may die young, leaving a family as yet unable to care for itself without her. Neglect and abuse of such orphaned children can shorten their lives, too, and such a natural 'culling' protects the continuance of those family units with fewer members.

In countries where the vagina is customarily in use early in puberty or in the teens, the life expectancy for women has always been low. Woman can die in their forties from overwork in caring for their offspring or from reproductive system disorders. The idea of having several wives per husband was sensible. It gave each wife less daily work and with each pregnancy, lactation usually meant no sex either. Prostitution also had its uses – wives were less used for sexual pleasure and the life of a prostitute was often short.

It can then be seen from this very brief look at history that too much sex may not necessarily be a good thing for women, just as trying to imitate men by wearing jeans and trousers is not good for female genital health. The body will at some point say, no!

At the moment, the 1980s show a huge growth in the numbers of old people, with many more women in their eighties than men. These particular generations have spent their youth *without* sexual permissiveness. The sheath was new, the Pill, coil and more modern contraceptives unused. The war took away much of their active sexual years and shortage of money meant less leisure for sexual activity. But at the end of their lives modern science has moved ahead of them and such drugs as antibiotics, diuretics and ventilators prolong or abort earlier attempts by the body to end its own life. Those particular women have lived a very long time. Gynaecological care is at the moment not good enough to match up to the modern, prolonged and frequent genito–urinary troubles of women. There is malpractice in many cases, which may help remove life quality and shorten life expectancy.

In my opinion we need to adjust the care of the female body. Where gynaecological care was previously insufficient because it didn't necessarily matter, it matters now in view of the acceptance of increased sexual activity and longevity. This new care must start before play-group and not cease even in old age. The quality of old age and genital health is more important since we are unfortunately going to be 'helped' to stay alive longer. If we don't care, we may live mentally and physically miserable existances, unfulfilled and probably with a shorter life expectancy, one much nearer the old norm.

Many cogs fit one wheel and I am a cog that promotes and teaches better care of the modern female genito-urinary system.

So if at the heart of the ordinary woman's idea of caring about the health of her reproductive organs there is something called the vagina, let's learn a little about how it works.

The Vagina in a child or a virgin is flat with all the sides touching. Only at the loss of virginity, on the first penile penetration, does it open up to become a round tunnel. This tunnel or passage has the cervix at the top and the vulva at the bottom.

The Hymen, at the vulval end of the vagina, is a fibrous area of tissue mainly there to protect children and young girls from infections. It is usually broken easily enough by penile penetration, but in some girls can be too tough and needs surgical help to break. There are also some hymens which are too elastic and, whilst allowing intercourse, can be nicked or split only to mend again. Such hymens may finally rupture during childbirth but usually intercourse itself is sufficiently sore to necessitate careful surgery. A hymen, if there's just too much of it, can limit the flow of menstrual blood and be responsible for low pain and swelling, so any girl starting periods and incapacitated by them should, for this and a variety of other reasons, be taken to a gynaecologist. I once read somewhere that virginity is the only object to become useful once you've lost it!

The Vulva is the medical name given to the area which we commonly call 'bottom'. It's an overall title which incorporates all the other named parts and openings. This whole area is rich in blood vessels, having arteries and veins interconnecting all over the place. It has numerous lymph glands which connect down both sides of the vulva but don't cross over to the thighs. The supremely sensitive nerve supply runs from the clitoris right along to the anus.

Because of the three openings in the vulva lying so near to one another, they can frequently affect one another. Internally also they are closely situated.

In front of the vaginal opening on the vulva is the urethral opening. This opening leads into the urethra, a little hollow tube which goes up into the bottom of the bladder. Urine rests in the bladder having journeyed there from the kidneys down two tubes called ureters, until you want to let it out.

Towards the back is the anal opening where waste body solids emerge as faeces. *These wastes are a major cause of infection of the vulva, vagina and urethra.*

The Cervix is up at the top of the vagina. It should be thought of really as the end of the uterus not the end of the vagina. The uterus/womb needs a really substantial and fleshy base for supporting a growing foetus and for protecting the baby's head in the last month or so of pregnancy. The cervix is comprised of part fibre, part muscle and has tremendous reserves of strength and elasticity for pushing the baby out. Around the time of ovulation, due to cyclical hormonal changes, the mucous membrane of the cervix manufactures and holds a little plug of liquid. This liquid lines the cervical canal and is an additional nourishment for travelling sperm when ejected in intercourse. It is alkaline and full of carbohydrate to encourage sperm on their amazing journey upwards to the Fallopian tubes and ripe eggs.

Near one part of the cervix, there is only about half an inch distance between it and the ureters leading down into the bladder. When a penis is introduced into the vagina and working in thrusting movements, it isn't just the cervix and vagina that have to cope with it, the rest of the surrounding tissue is there to help reduce bruising of other nearby organs like the ureters, bladder and bowels.

This tissue padding is caused not only by eating and drinking sufficiently for a reasonable weight, its amount is also dictated by hormone activity. Oestrogens and progestogens play a major part in the workings of the reproductive system and will be dealt with later on. Through the centre of the cervix runs a canal. Each month

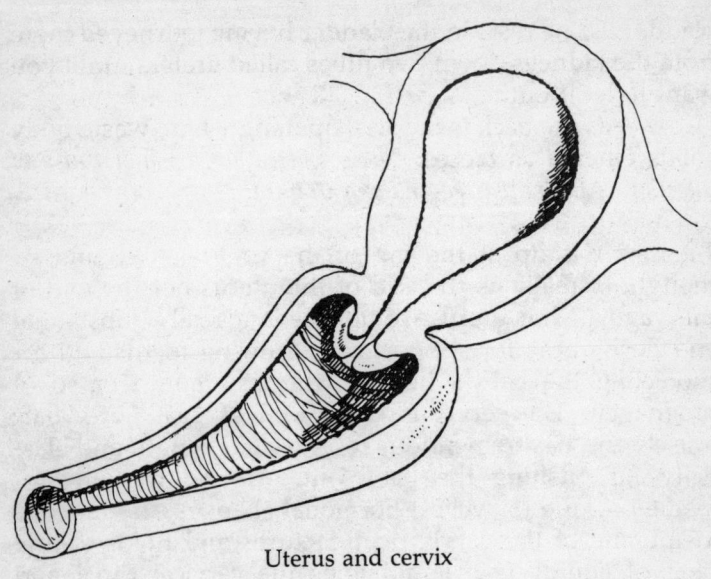

Uterus and cervix

menstrual blood comes down it into the vagina and a baby, too, uses the canal to come through when it is born.

The Uterus/Womb is about three and a half inches long and in most women tilts forward so that it lies over the top of the bladder. It has muscle, about one inch thick. This muscle stretches with the developing foetus and then after birth sinks back, although a bit floppy now, into something near its former size. The width of the uterus is about two and a half inches but this can vary greatly and the length of the hollow cavity from the top to the start of the cervix is about three inches. The uterus is extremely strong and extremely flexible, and exercising it back to shape after birth is greatly recommended. The uterus has a lining called the endometrium, a brilliant piece of organisation on nature's part. This lining is constantly growing and then being discarded. It consists of rich blood oozing out

36

of the walls of the uterus, which are thick with blood vessels, and roughly every twenty-eight days it drops off and comes through the cervix, down the vagina and onto whatever sanitary protection you choose. There are several reasons why it may not drop off, but if you are sexually active and *not* using contraception, the chances are that there's a fertilized egg attaching itself to the endometrium for nourishment on the rich blood and that a baby will emerge through the cervix and vagina some nine months later. Menstrual bleeding starts at puberty, in the early teens and usually finishes with the menopause after the age of forty-five.

The uterus is an upside down pear-shape, the stalk being the cervix and the flat fleshy part being the top. Into the top of the uterus lead two openings or tubes called the Fallopian tubes and it is in these that the swimming sperms encounter eggs which their instincts tell them to fertilize. Eggs come from both of the two ovaries, which manufactured them many years in advance and now expel a small number each monthly cycle. Unfertilized eggs continue on from the Fallopian tubes into the uterus, where they get washed out of the body in each monthly bleed.

Let's just look at the vagina in detail. Recently a gynaecologist said to me that the medical profession didn't think too much about the vagina 'because it wasn't of great medical interest.' Isn't this quite contrary to the views of the female patient? We find our vaginas thoroughly fascinating! And what would men and male gynaecologists think if vaginas were to be removed overnight the world over? What about their pleasurable penile thrusting, and what about the introduction of sperm for the continuance of the human race? I tell you, I'm sure vaginas would be elevated to a newer level of interest.

Women are quite attached to their vaginas. They are pleasurable and comforting: sources of harmony when the

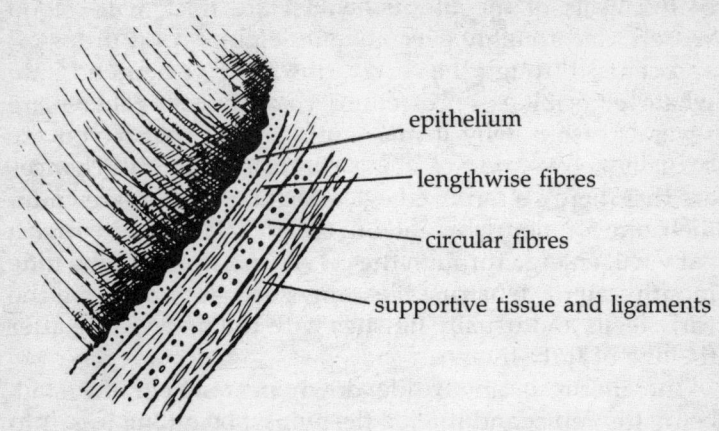

epithelium

lengthwise fibres

circular fibres

supportive tissue and ligaments

Layers of the vagina

day has been fractious, sources of annoyance when they are too dry or too runny, sources of pain during and after childbirth, or sources of swelling and soreness after sex. Women need to 'know' their vaginas and learn to live with them. Do *you* know *your* vagina?

Like the uterus, the vagina also needs to be extremely elastic. The walls are a basic mixture of fibre and muscle, the first layer of which has lengthwise fibres and the second layer circular fibres. The skin that you can touch in the vagina is called the epithelium and it has several layers before the fibre/muscle sections begin. The epithelial surface is moist and constantly shedding itself in the form of cells. The cells are washed away in the moisture which carries a number of other things like glycogen, lactobacilli and hormones, particularly oestrogen.

If you have enough lactobacilli, the vaginal pH (levels of acidity and alkalinity) stays at around 4.5 – mildly acidic – and fends off most low bacterial invasions from the vulva including thrush (monilia). In children, before puberty,

38

there's no glycogen and no lactobacilli which makes the vaginal pH around 7.0–7.5 and alkaline. The glycogen decreases after menopause with a corresponding drop in lactobacilli and acidity making the vagina again alkaline.

Beyond the circular muscle fibres at the outer layers of the vagina are layers of supportive skin tissue and ligaments to hold the tissues in place. The major blood vessel is the vaginal artery, supplying blood to the vaginal area, and used blood is carried away from the area by the branches and trunk of the iliac vein. The whole lower pelvic area, most particularly the vulva and its openings, are heavily supplied with tiny blood vessels and nerve endings for sexual excitement and reproductive fuctions, which need a lot of strength for muscular activity during labour.

The Pelvic Floor Muscles as you can see from the diagram, are a web-like network of incredible strength. They literally stop your internal organs from falling out. It you lose some of their strength, as after childbirth, there may be

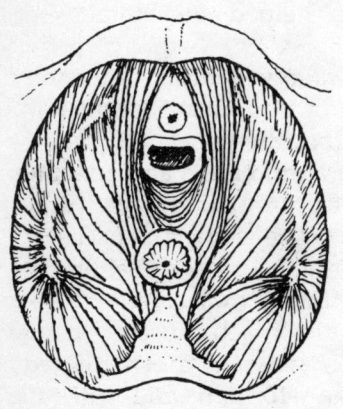 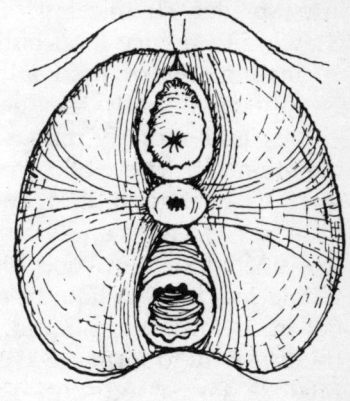

Muscle cross section   Muscle tissue layer

great nuisance effects of poor bladder control, bowel control or lowering of the uterus called prolapse. Regular lifelong exercises will maintain and regain their strength. Each and every day of your life when you pull up, push down, push out, sit in a chair and so on, this network of muscles is at work commanded by the trillions of nerve endings that connect, through the spinal column, into bigger ones within the brain.

To protect, pad out and tidy up these superb muscles there is a good layer of supportive skin tissue which is a mixture of smoother fibre and finer muscle.

Part of the pelvic floor, the back part or perineum, contains the anus, from which faeces emerge, and it is worth a minute or two of time to revise the system with which our body digests the food we eat, because the bacteria which our bodies grow and use for mulching this food are the very ones which can cause so much sexual cystitis.

The tastiness of any food we eat acts to stimulate the salivary glands in our mouth. In saliva is an enzyme called ptyalin which starts straight away to break down the food into smaller chemical groups, helped considerably by chewing to reduce food bulk.

Small pieces of food are swallowed down the gullet (oesophagus) with the help of muscular contraction, gravity and slippery mucus. From the gullet, food enters the stomach, where all sorts of amino acids and enzymes start to change it into specific groups of fats, carbohydrates, proteins and vitamins. The stomach muscles act like a Mouli or Kenwood Mixer and for a while churn the whole mess into a liquidy mixture of molecules. When it becomes sufficiently liquid, the stomach muscles change their activity to form a wave-like action so that the liquidy mixture is passed out of the stomach and into the duodenum which is about ten inches in length.

As the acids and enzymes continue working on the

molecules of what was once delicious food and drink, but is becoming a brown mess, those molecules become so small that they can actually be absorbed through the lining of the duodenum and small intestine into the bloodstream. The molecules are carried by the bloodstream to the liver and elsewhere so that the proteins, fats, minerals and vitamins necessary for our healthy muscles, blood, bones, hair, teeth etc. are used. The unnecessary molecules continue their journey into the large intestine.

The small intestine is about twenty feet long and is bacteria-free, but the large intestine, about five foot long, contains millions of bacteria. The walls are very muscular in order to push the food molecules along their inevitable route, spending a few hours in the small intestine and a day or so in the large intestine.

In the large intestine, additional enzymes, acids and now bacteria continue to emulsify the remaining molecules of fats, minerals, carbohydrates, proteins and vitamins which the body's natural balancing and weighing has rejected as being unnecessary. After some time the emulsified waste reforms into the shape of the colon or bowel and becomes faeces. These vary in width, length and shape according to what food or drugs you have eaten. *All faeces, whether liquid or hard, are absolutely teeming with germs. Inside the bowel they are quite harmless, but outside they can kill if the circumstances are right, and they can cause all sorts of health variations up to that. If you get bacterial cystitis, this last paragraph should be read carefully again.*

If we are to complete the 'et al' in a chapter entitled 'The Vagina Et Al', we must include the urethral opening and its function.

This book is entitled *Sexual Cystitis* and if the vagina represents the sexual, so the urethral opening with its higher connecting urinary system of the bladder, ureters and kidneys must represent the cystitis. The urethral opening lies between the clitoris and vagina. The clitoris is the sensitive gland which brings on sexual arousal in foreplay. From its actual opening, the urethral tube, or urethra, rises one and a half inches into the bladder. The surface of the tube, over which urine runs as it's being passed out, is made up of layers of skin and epithelium, and is backed by tissue. There are muscle fibres, mostly coiled around like a spring, but some running lengthwise in a connection with similar ones in the bladder, so that the passing of urine is designed to be a co-ordinated effort between these two sorts of muscles.

The back wall of the urethra lies extremely close to the front wall of the vagina and consequently anything inserted into the vagina temporarily displaces, flattens or massages the urethral walls whilst it's there. A full understanding of this fact is extremely important in any dealings with sexual cystitis.

The top end of the urethra leads up into the bladder. The bladder is a collecting vessel for waste body fluids. Its great convenience to its owner lies in the fact that it works only to command and intention rather than dribbling out all the time. When something like two or three hundred millilitres of urine has been accumulated, the bladder sends out signals that micturition is now desirable and necessary. So the nearest loo is sought, the pelvic floor muscles loosen, and up in the bladder walls, which are also aided by other muscles in the abdominal walls, downward contractions start to allow urine to escape down the urethra and out into the lavatory pan.

The bladder itself is made of loose muscles which allow it to expand and contract according to the amount of urine inflowing from the two ureters on either side of its top surface. Part of it lies very close to the front walls of the womb and the bottom part is directly lying on the front part of the cervix.

These expansive muscles are covered by a rough mucous membrane which becomes much smoother and stronger near the internal end of the urethra. This smooth area of membrane is called the trigone, and it acts like the strengthened base of a bowl in order to bear the weight and pressure of gathering urine.

In the top of the bladder are two openings which each lead into the ureter. Each of the two ureters are about ten inches long and have a one-way valve at the bottom end which allows collected droplets of urine to pass just one way – downwards into the bladder. At the higher end of each they fatten out a bit into a funnel-shaped thing called the renal pelvis. This further enlarges and becomes the kidney.

We each have two kidneys about the size of a medium cupped hand. They are an inch to an inch and a half thick, measure about four and a half inches from top to bottom and maybe two and a half inches wide. They are a wonder of nature.

The blood supply of each is connected up to the other by the main artery and vein of the body. Arteries carry blood *to* organs from the heart, and veins carry it *away* from organs back to the heart. The artery that branches out of the big main body artery, or aorta, is called the renal artery and the vein that branches off the big main body vein into the kidneys is called the inferior vena cava.

The renal arteries into each kidney carry about fifteen continuously flowing gallons of blood an hour – that's how busy the kidneys are – and the inferior vena cava carries it all out again. In that blood is carried all the minerals, salts, proteins, amino acids, vitamins and fats that our small intestines absorbed into their walls and on into the bloodstream.

So here is the big link up with what we eat and drink. An astonishing number of functions are performed by each kidney, but we'll stick, or try to stick, to that one which ends up as the urine which so interests us here in this book.

The renal artery branches out into estuaries of finer arteries called capillaries. The estuaries – which are minute – are enclosed in capsules. Mr Bowman discovered them and named them after himself, so they are Bowman's capsules. Each capsule collects water out of the blood and disperses it into a narrow tube called a renal tubule. Here something happens to condense the amount of water into an even smaller, stronger amount and then it passes into other tubules which send the newly formed liquid called urine into the renal pelvis out down the ureter. When enough urine collects in the bottom end of the ureter, the sphincter valve there opens to let it down into the bladder.

Urine is basically made of waste proteins called urea, but there is also some salt, body acids from the act of digestion, uric acid and water. The waste particles of carbohydrates and fats finally leave the body as carbon dioxide which our lungs breathe out, and not via the urine.

The colouring of normal yellow urine is made with urochrome, which science doesn't know much about as yet, and other variations in colour are caused mostly by the amount of liquid we have drunk. Drink too little and urine is more acid and browner in colour, drink a lot and it is much paler and doesn't sting.

Normal urine is slightly acid, but the acidity levels can be varied by our daily liquid consumption. If protein is shown in a urine test it indicates a possible infection. If sugar is found in urine it may mean the bloodstream has been overloaded with a heavy sugar intake or it could also mean you are diabetic and have an insulin disorder.

Urine samples are taken for aiding the correct diagnosis of many illnesses and are as important as blood samples.

In addition to what you drink and the amount of it, there is a sensitive organ in a gland in the base of the brain which reacts to the amount of water currently in the bloodstream. This organ is responsible for the releasing of the amounts of special hormone that is anti-diuretic. A diuretic substance makes you pass lots of urine, an *anti*-diuretic *restricts* the amount you pass. This anti-diuretic hormone is manufactured by the pituitary gland, which is also the seat of sexuality and links up to infrequent urination during pre-mentrual tension. The anti-diuretic hormone reduces the urine excreted by persuading the renal tubules not to discard the water from the bloodstreams but to hold on to it.

There is so much interlinking of systems within the renal functions that whole books can, and have, been written by specialists. Progress in understanding is still continuing and I don't feel we need dwell longer here for our purposes, but knowing the background to urine production is important.

I have given slightly more information in these descriptions of reproductive and renal organs than in my other books because I do feel that we, as patients, need to upgrade our knowledge in order to help ourselves. Yet, let us not forget that much of this knowledge is nothing more than simple high school examination level which, presumably, not many of us bothered to take in.

If you need to get to grips with cystitis, now's the time to comprehend some of its background.

PART ONE

Preparation for Intercourse

Sizes and Scars

Preparation for intercourse should involve *two* people – both the man and the woman. We haven't discussed the male and his internal organs because it's not usually him who gets the cystitis. He could well develop any one of several nasty transmittable diseases and have urinary discomfort as a by-product, but he certainly has little knowledge of what it's like to have a full-blown attack of cystitis within forty-eight hours of intercourse.

However, since a man is one half of the act of intercourse let's try to understand him a little better. Without boring ourselves into madness, we must by now all know that his spermatozoa – sperm – are ejaculated all round and over the cervix during orgasm.

These millions of sperms swim through the cervical canal into the uterus and up into the Fallopian tubes where just one of their number, out of all those millions, attacks and impregnates one egg to fertilize it. The egg can remain as one or divide up for twins, triplets, quads etc.

This is fine if you want a baby, but the burden of a large unwanted family can be just as great for the average man as for the average woman. His income could never support all the babies he could be capable of making from puberty, and so the majority of thinking men look for some way of breaking nature's neat reproductive system.

Male writers on sex tend to gloss over the male organ. They matter of factly mention its length in minimum and maximum measurements, but seem generally to impart that whatever size it is, it's the greatest wonder-entertainer that woman has! How lucky she is, we all hear, and it is what he does *with* it that's more important than its size! Well, that may be true but if men are going to learn the real truth they must first understand that not one of them is identical in shape, size or feel to a woman. A young man in his twenties is too thin to fully pleasure a woman in her thirties after two or three children; he is also almost too hard when fully erect for a younger woman's comfort. Some men 'leak' from the penis during foreplay which may mean to them or their doctor that they're fertile but may make oral foreplay a bit undesirable to some women.

I have yet to meet a woman who thinks the sight of an approaching erect penis is beautiful! It isn't a pretty sight! It's an essential sight – true – and she probably feels quite pleased that he can be aroused by just looking at her and knowing that he will be allowed to go the whole way to orgasm.

Foreskins are funny to some women, but when it boils down to it, what our partner has is what we've got to put up with! If he's there with a floppy foreskin whose cleanliness is not number one on his list of preparations, you had better do something about it. Be artful, try working a warm bath into the preamble so that you can get in too and work him over a bit with some soap. Only use a pure soap – nothing scented, cheap, antiseptic or deodorised or you'll swell up the penis unbearably. As you soap it for him pull back the foreskin and give the thing a damn good clean up and rinse off. He'll absolutely love this and be half-drowning himself up the far end, both in the bath water and his own ecstasy.

If the occasion doesn't readily present itself for ablutions then your other resort is to request an early wearing of the sheath, which is not so dreaded now because of improvements in the quality of the latex and plastic compounds. Sheaths are enjoying a revival because they are the cleanest and most effective way of preventing sexual illness. Every woman should carry one and every man should carry several.

Fingernails are a good outward sign of any inward bent to hygiene. Look at his hands and nails and get a feel for the ingrained dirt both on the hands, fingertips and around and under the nails themselves. Are they jagged or too long? Obviously balance this with the job he does: you can't expect a motor mechanic to look as though he was the chairman of the Stock Exchange. Not that the desk-bound man can afford to be proud. He's often too thoughtless or lazy to wash after work at the office when he's arrived home, having read the paper and opened the train doors that everyone else touches.

I once counselled a middle-aged American woman in one of Jeddah's big company compounds and, after many questions, then spent time on her husband's hygiene. Although he washed his hands in the washroom before coming home, the oils from his job as a rig supervisor and site lecturer needed a second removal effort at home in the compound house. So he reached for the washing up liquid *and* the heavy duty Swarfega every night. All her urine results were negative over the seventeen years of her marriage, which had been blighted with cystitis. Her husband had always worked in the oil industry and they always had plenty of foreplay – a feature they both loved. The oils and oil removers were ingrained on his hands. He wasn't skin sensitive but she was.

If your regular sexual partner cannot get his foreskin back down the penis sit him down, give him several stiff drinks, tell him that the bacteria in your urine sample could be from similar ones trapped under his foreskin. Tell him sex feels uncomfortable, too, as the foreskin may be preventing his smooth entry into your vagina. Persuade him to see a really good genito-urinary specialist and explain the sexual situation so that swabs of the mucous under the foreskin can be taken and analysed. If these do match up with your own bacterial results, you'd better sit him down again and get him really high so that he agrees to having circumcision in as anaesthetised a way as possible!

A circumsised man can be two things to two women. One woman can revel in the firmness and cleanness of his thrusts in and out of her vagina but a different woman with a tighter vagina could be bruised by that same firmness and rigidity. The uncircumcised man with his foreskin intact might be able to put this extra padding to good use as a shock absorber so that the sensitive vagina would receive a more muted force.

Thin-skinned or thinly-padded epithelial lining in the vagina is easily traumatized so that for instance, diet-ridden women beneath the hundred and twelve pound weight mark (eight stone), or anorexics, find every act of intercourse a really miserable event. They don't lubricate properly, they can't tolerate more than a few minutes of intercourse without feeling sore. This vaginal soreness rapidly affects the equally thin muscles and fibres of the urethra which lie, as we know from the previous chapter, right in front of the vagina.

Let's look at penile length and vaginal length. It's often bandied around, especialy by men, that short men don't necessarily have a short penis, likewise tall men a long penis, but I'd approach that information with some scepticism. Bar the usual exceptions to any case, I'd say from a woman's eye view that indeed short men do tend on the whole to have shorter organs than taller men.

I believe that nature helps satisfy both sexes by mating or pairing up the majority of short men with short women, tall men with tall women and all the variations of size in between. A short woman, say five feet tall would, even with a good elastic vagina, be most unlikely to have comfortable intercourse with a man six foot two, and vice versa a short man to a tall woman.

The vagina can stretch tremendously but the actual length from entrance to cervix doesn't alter in intercourse nearly as much as the width, so if there's a length problem in any given sexual partnership the cervix is just going to be badly battered at each coupling and throughout the duration of each coupling. Right in front of the cervix and the cervical canal is the base of the bladder. Even if little urine is in there during the spell of time that intercourse takes place, that bladder is certainly going to be pummelled like bread dough. If the bladder hasn't been totally emptied before intercourse it's going to feel like a rolling waterbed or loose jelly with a thumb being poked in and out of it. The urine inside the bladder will be like a shield fending off bricks and stones, something for the bladder wall and the cervix to be banged against during intercourse.

It's more often true that short men make up in width what they may lack in length, so some women may not only have no length bruising but may benefit from the extra sensations of pleasure from penile width. If she's too thinly padded, though, she'll still be in trouble. The same can be true for people of other height – the pairs do need to match their sexual organs for excitement, comfort and reward.

In the years before science took infertility seriously, women were frequently 'assessed' for marriage by 'good child-bearing hips' because a rounded and wide pelvis was thought to be a good sign of ready child-bearing and easy birthing. Not that this was foolproof, but certainly still today with the modern monitoring of labour, doctors do measure the foetal head in relation to the pelvic floor. If the head is larger, then they have to deliver by Caesarian section.

The head may pass through the cervical canal and vaginal canal all right, but the actual vaginal opening may be very badly stressed. If there's time, enough maternal energy left and a patient medical staff it can be nice to keep pushing and stretching, but if factors are adverse, the hated and sometimes quite unnecessary episiotomy is performed. The doctor cleanly slits the vaginal opening backwards with a scalpel rather than let it tear. A jagged tear is more difficult to sew than a straight cut.

Every woman who has had an episiotomy knows it, and feels it to have left a much weaker perineum. The scarline can harbour infection more readily and can often nick or split on intercourse if she's not really careful. Penetration must be gentle and the entire shaft of the penis lubricated as well as inside the vagina. If injury does occur and any bacteria are present on the perineal skin then a blood-borne infection can begin. The scar, either of a natural tear or of a medical episiotomy, takes ages to heal after birth because that area is seldom absolutely dry. Mucous from the vagina, from sweating, from droplets of urine and faecal farting make the perineum quite a moist area.

This moisture readily promotes soreness and bacteria and prevents early recovery from injury. An episiotomy can delay the resumption of intercourse after birth by three or four months and can also make the simple act of sitting down comfortably an extremly uncomfortable business. Women suffer in silence from the after-effects of an episiotomy but doctors should know that we don't like it.

It isn't only external scarring that can have a detrimental effect on intercourse. Almost worse are the unseen injuries to the vagina and cervix that have healed badly because doctors tend to leave them unexplored and unchecked. Unless they are actually looked for they can't be sewn up properly. The cervix may not go fully back to its normal size and remain a degree or two dilated. It may have a tear which is extremely painful when the head of the penis bangs it and splits it again. Bacteria will invade the blood vessels ruptured in the split and there could be much repeated suffering with a not unnatural loss of libido. If you feel that you have not seen a diminution of sexual discomfort in the six months following childbirth, or if you have a regular point of soreness or pain inside, this must be reported to a gynaecologist. If the first one fails to find the reason then look for a second opinion and go on searching until some gynaecologist does find a cause for the trouble. No matter how small he says the reason is – it's not his pain, go ahead and request him to repair whatever he has found. A lot of lifelong damage can be done in childbirth.

Not all hymens break easily at the first attempt at inter-course. Most girls are extremely apprehensive about the first effort by a man to put his penis inside her. You can read a hundred books about what it feels like and what the mechanics are, but it's still like any 'first time' in life when you yourself actually experience it. Every single woman remembers the occasion in detail – the room, the man, the state of the sheets and the feeling of being opened up.

Men, too, remember their first ejaculation or their first penetration of a girl and where they did it. It's still a bit of a feather in their cap to break a hymen, even these days.

With such natural apprehension and maybe the awkwardness of failure the first time, go at it for the second time with two or three strong painkillers and a good dollop of lubricating jelly like KY Jelly by Johnson and Johnson. If this and other attempts prove unrewarding and miserable, it's no good carryuing on so go to a gynaecologist. He will assess the toughness of the hymen and decide whether a local or general anaesthetic will be required for the operation to break it. It should be carefully removed and tied up, or jagged flaps of it will make intercourse sore and bloody. You could be laying yourself up for years of trouble with an impeded vaginal entrance so it will pay to sort it all out at the start.

I must end such a section by begging the reader to take out private health insurance from an early adult age because so many sad ladies find their way to me for counselling in utter despair. The State health services are not always reliable and before gynaeological trouble sets in (if it does) that is the time to take out insurance. If you do it once you have become ill, that illness will not be acceptable to the health insurance company.

Desires, Despairs and Diseases

Desire for intercourse! How do you know if you desire intercourse? If you are a man your penis swells up and throbs, if you're a woman your vagina secretes a varying amount of sticky, wet, clear mucous which is a preparatory lubricant for aiding entry of a penis inside you.

The desire for it is an inherent part of any species of life on this planet for the purpose of the continuity of that species. There's absolutely nothing that can be done to alter this fact. The vast majority of humans follow this desire to greater or lesser degrees of action. A minority have no desire to mate in this way but choose to explore their bisexual, homosexual or lesbian characteristics.

The vast majority doesn't want a baby each time intercourse happens but the sexual desire is equally intense and grows over the years of prime sexual activity. It starts to decrease slowly as middle age wears on into later years, although men can remain fertile far longer than women whose child-bearing abilities cease when menstrual periods stop around the late forties and early fifties.

All manner of stimulus can set off the desire to be sexually active. I've mentioned already music, dancing, clothing, perfume, advertisements or films of erotic images and erotic or pornographic writing. Perhaps a quiet field in the sun, or a poolside littered with brown oily bodies, reminiscences of previous sex acts, attentive fellow travellers, or the Trooping of the Colour with two thousand guardsmen rhythmically pounding around Horse Guards Parade on the Queen's Birthday will get you going!

If you are lucky enough to be in a stimulating, responsive and healthy sexual liaison, then the delight of knowing gazes and touches of tensing nipples and penis create a very special bond. It's a bond that grows and with time will become unforgettable. Recalling times and places, even when parted, can be exciting enough to put the vagina into delicate and exquisite spasm only relieved by self-help. Few actively sexual men can withstand their own version of this tension without their own preferred alleviation of it.

If you are unlucky enough to be in a stimulating, responsive but *unhealthy* sexual liaison you know what frustration, desperation and discomfort is. To want intercourse with the man of your desire and for him to want you too, but to know that the fulfilment is denied because sex is in some way, either during or after, responsible for soreness, discomfort and pain is to know the bottom of a deep, deep well of unhappiness.

When you can't seem to put it right and the doctor is sick of the sight of you, it is only natural to go off the whole business. This leads to unbearable tensions, rows and anger and only worsens the situation. Up and down the country there are many sexual relationships in this misery, so eat that as a mere crumb of comfort. My own husband, worrying about his part in my suffering, took himself off to have intercourse with another woman apparently to prove to himself, not me because I wasn't told about it for some years, that he wasn't the cause.

There was no fault on his part but quite decidedly, the iron ramrod that is most young men can be very unyielding to the unbirthed vagina and the tight muscle

58

fibres of the pelvic floor. Like a new spring, the ability to expand is certainly there but a fully extended stretch hasn't yet eased the fine new tension. Plenty of lubrication is what's needed and a willingness to recognize the limitations of the novice vagina.

And sex is a trouble-laden exercise. The bowels of both men and women are teeming with billions of potentially lethal bacteria and whether a penis or a finger is inserted there, it will come out absolutely coated with faecal deposit. The fingernail will gather it up in the quick and under the nail itself so that the very next thing touched will be contaminated whether it's the sheet, the lavatory flush, the basin tap or any part of its owner or sexual partner.

To then move such a contaminated finger along a female perineum and caress the clitoris or work into the vagina is as good as stuffing her with cow dung. The resulting infections will put her out of sexual activity for three to four weeks. Aids has pulled up many men whether they be bisexual, homosexual or wayward heterosexual, and it has pointed out quite clearly that if you attempt to use the wrong area of the body for sex you could pay with your life.

Before any woman lets her desire for intercourse run away with her senses, it could be vital to try to assess a new man's sexuality. If you've a doubt about him possibly being bisexual ask with whom he lives, what his hobbies are, where and with whom did he holiday last time. When closeness is gaining on you both, ask him outright if he likes anal sex. If he shudders, you're safe, if he says 'now and again', go to the ladies and leave by the back door! There are plenty of other men around.

It is essential when sleeping casually that you insist on your partner using the sheath. It's your life that could be at stake, not his temporary pleasure. The Aids virus outbreak must now show the truth of that. Don't forget that you are not his first-ever woman, because once he's into his twenties there may have been strings of casual vaginas that he has used.

Aids is not the only resulting disease of casual intercourse. Antibiotics have inhibited the spreading of gonorrhoea and syphilis, but there are other very troublesome infections that are transmitted in intercourse when not prevented by the physical barrier of a condom.

The additional problem of these infections is that they can also spring up at any time even between faithful partners. Your own body, under all sorts of conditions favourable to differing bacteria, can start a problematical discharge, soreness, dryness and infection all by itself.

Just having one of these problems in your own sexual organs making you feel low and having to forgo sexual release is quite bad enough. Passing it on to the boyfriend or husband is often secondary in your thoughts to your own pain, itchiness, back-ache, discharge or whatever. Frequent bouts of something like thrush can really get you to screaming pitch. Unexplained vaginal discharges create hair-pulling, head-banging sessions of great despair.

No-one, but no-one, can fully appreciate life-long memories of wrecked holidays and outings on which, to all outward appearances, you and your partner are in seventh heaven when inwardly you are both enduring such precious times without natural sexual release. Hand and oral sex, whilst useful substitutes, may create even more tension and need for release. Nothing can really beat the great finalities of full male and female orgasm.

The medications these days for cystitis and vaginal illnesses are much improved, having shorter dosages with diminished side effects, but it is hateful to have to keep going back to the doctor when yet another bout starts. Each time you always think it's the last. You try so hard to get a positive attitude and put the past behind you. Each time you're wrong, you search and search for the cure. Your sexual partner tries hard to be patient seeing your tears, but inevitably his own sexual frustration wells up and you start arguing. Maybe you put all care aside and fling yourself into his arms for lovemaking which is too fast for satisfaction, imperils the early effectiveness of the medication and lengthens the duration of the trouble still further.

Every discharge or reddened vulva can be different from the previous one, so don't make the mistake of telling your doctor you've got 'X' again when it *may* now be 'Y' if it's put under a microscope. Never take it for granted that you have another attack of thrush: it could be a heavy hormonal discharge of the vaginal epithelial cells which can be equally irritating and thick.

You must, probably against difficult local odds, try to get a vaginal examination and swabs. The swabs should be pain-free – after all they're only long cotton buds – and taken from the cervix, the middle vagina and the vulva. I really cannot think why small pathology labs aren't available for sample testing of all sorts in big towns. If doctors expect women to insert medicated treatment pessaries, why aren't we trustworthy enough to take a simple high vaginal swab? I am well aware that without a speculum it isn't possible to take three separate swabs because the speculum props open the vaginal walls enabling a clean 'take' from the cervix. But when you think of the hollow applicators used with vaginal medicated creams, it ought to be feasible to have a home-use kit on that line for clean taking of swabs.

I once did this in Lagos where virtually anything goes and you can buy the appropriate treatment without prescription. The fuss it saved, the time and anguish it saved! One really does get fed up with some of the red tape practised in modern western medicine.

Trichomonas

This is a parasite which loves to live in moist areas. It can be transmitted from male to female and vice versa during intercourse, therefore behaving like a ping-pong ball. Once inside the vagina it lives within the mucous secretions, or even on the wall of the vagina. Occasionally it can sink further into the epithelium and get a good hold between the cells. If your male partner is carrying the trichomonal bacteria, he won't know it because he is usually symptom free but if you have it, he almost certainly will too.

The first obvious sign of trich is vaginal flooding, feeling much like a heavy period when you stand up after sitting down, except that the flooding isn't blood, it is brownish, frothy, smelly and can literally run down your legs. This discharge is wickedly irritating and if you look at the pictures you'll shudder to see the swimming ability of all its flagella. Trich is built to live in water – that is its habitat.

If you don't at first recognize that this is a special discharge you soon will, because as well as the first two mentioned symptoms worsening, another one will start to involve the urethra and make that sting. The stinging shortly becomes cystitis and you won't quite know what to do with yourself with a combination of stinging, flooding and irritation!

For heaven's sake don't be tempted by intercourse at such a time. The vulva, vagina, urethra et al will react most unfavourably! Go to a VD unit, special clinic or genito-urinary clinic where swabs will be taken and free treatment of oral tablets called Flagyl, dispensed. Trich will not abate with any other treatment. Flagyl comes in the form of an oral tablet rather than pessaries or creams because it passes through the secretions in the vagina and cervix and through the urinary system via the urine to reach all affected organs simultaneously.

When trich, albeit without symptoms, is in the long male urethra, it can reach the prostate gland and just keep on being transmitted into a woman through ejaculation. It is most important, therefore, that the man and woman are treated with the same drug, Flagyl, at the same time. At least one week of treatment is required, and you may need two. Trichomonal parasites die on contact with dry air so ideally the gynaecologist or family doctor should have a microscope in his room for quick recognition, but if a good smear of it is specially stained in a laboratory analysis then some of the dead trich will still show up.

Sometimes gonococcal bacteria are found to be linking up with trichomonal parasites, so a good smear and lab test is important. Gonococcal bacteria are relatively rare but when trichomonas is present, because of absent hygiene or regular promiscuity, it is wise to check also for gonorrhoea which arises under similar conditions.

If gonorrhoea remains undiscovered, the bacteria will thoroughly infect the cervix, swim up the cervical canal past the uterus and on into the Fallopian tubes. Once embedded here gonococcal infection will add high fever, nausea and pain to your discharge symptoms and inflame the wall of the tubes. If the tubes swell up you may eventually become infertile.

The safest and most effective treatment from gonorrhoea is injected penicillin but obviously something else would have to be used if penicillin disagrees with you.

Something Completely Innocent

Leaving two of the 'heavies' for a moment let's look at something completely innocent. It bugged me for at least one full year and may well have been doing so on and off over the years.

I can't remember doing so, but at some point, I have

changed from white bread to brown like so many people. My bowels have always been their own master since childhood and undoubtedly were more solid in the days of thick and frequent slices of white bread for tea at my mother's home. On marriage, tea gave way to a cooked meal, but in my years abroad, brown bread still hadn't been adopted so I can only think that this problem I'm about to describe only began as recently as 1982.

The bowels are stimulated by bran to act more smoothly and no-one ever seems to understand that it doesn't run a beacon path *just* to the bowels. It could, as I already knew, overload the urine as well and agitate the bladder to work more often, but it never dawned on me that an effect might also be felt via the vaginal mucus.

None of the doctors I saw, and who took swabs, found any bacteria at all in what was almost as profuse a clear discharge as trichomonas. The anal opening was always wet, the vulva was wet and the whole perineum was very, very sore. The wetness alone was itchy though nothing like a bacterially infected discharge. No urinary symptoms ever developed.

I was very frustrated and anxious, especially since all swabs came up negative. Every gynaecologist said I should try to keep dry. How could I when I didn't know what the wetness was, or where, or why it was being produced?

As so much chance has it – a rare visit to a gynaecologist to whom I refer 'difficult' women – entailed some general checks on myself looking for nothing in particular. On palpating (feeling) my abdomen he said that he thought I was eating too much fibre. I didn't think I was because I know it upsets me, but I totted up the amount of brown wholemeal bread I had eaten the day before and got to six or seven slices – two for breakfast, two in a sandwich for lunch, one with toast and honey for tea because it was a miserable day then bread again to mop up a stew!

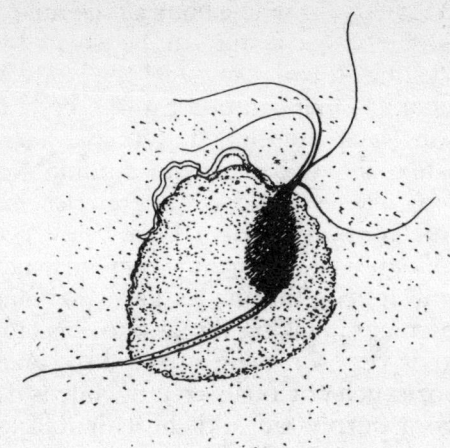

Trichomonas Vaginalis

For two days after the visit to him I cut out brown bread except for one slice of morning toast. The wetness that had driven me wild was disappearing in twenty-four hours and had gone in forty-eight hours. For the next few days, I remained absolutely dry. With interested experimenting over a couple of months I found that between one and three slices have no effect – over three and the anal opening moistens up so does the vagina.

I pass this on for interest and to remind everyone that so-called healthy living can be faddish and often *not* healthy for many people.

Candida Albicans

Let's look at a fungus by way of diversity. We all know it – vaginal thrush, of course, and it can be called candida albicans, yeast infection or monilia.

What most people – and I really mean most people, doctors included – fail to acknowledge is that candida albicans is a native of our whole body *all* the time. Candida albicans is also blood-borne and can be isolated in appropriate blood testing. It can also infest the bladder walls.

On given changes that can occur in the body for many variable reasons later mentioned, candida can upsurge. When the system is overloaded with candida it can erupt in the mouth as dryness, and white granules around the lips, palate and larynx. The vulva down below goes a dark purply-red and stiffens. The vagina may or may not ooze stringy, creamy mucus that itches like crazy and moves all over the perineum making things like episiotomy scars or haemorrhoids very sore. The anus is also contaminated but doesn't ooze such obviously creamy mucus. Labia also stiffen and go a purply-red and the hair follicles (roots) itch unmercifully as the fungus attacks them. At this picturesque point lie down on a clean towel on the floor with a good mirror and have a long look at yourself. It's useful to see it all looking thoroughly unhealthy so that there's a comparable yardstick for when its AOK.

Don't scratch it!

If you scratch it, like I did in the three solid years of antibiotics taken during my five years of cystitis in the late 'sixties, you too will have years of lichenized patches of labial skin that will irritate even on the brush of a petticoat.

Wash the discharge off quickly every few hours with a bottle of cool or cold water poured down the perineum whilst you sit on the loo. Dab it absolutely dry – really bone dry with kitchen towel, not loo paper because that will leave little bits behind. If you dry it with a cloth at this highly infective state the cloth will need to be changed each time so kitchen towel is probably the most sensible for a day or so.

Don't walk anywhere!

Sit down and sit back. Wear a long, loose skirt and no undies for maximum first aid and minimum spread of the discharge.

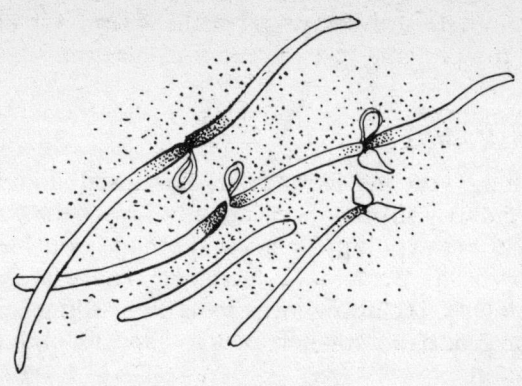

Candida bacteria

Thrush, under a microscope, looks like very fine spaghetti, tied or looped at intervals with thread. It is always wise to have a vaginal swab to confirm its presence because it is possible to have mild thrush without a readily seen discharge.

In terms of medical treatment, you will be given any one of a three to seven-day course of Gynodaktarin, Canesten or Nystatin pessaries or cream. Additionally, it would help to have oral Nystatin tablets or Nystatin boxed powder and certainly, if you ever have to have a course of antibiotics for something and are prone to thrush, you should take Nystatin tablets or powder as a preventative measure alongside the antibiotics.

The old gentian violet swabbing is infrequently used now, mostly because doctors are somewhat carefree in their attitude to vaginal work, but also because gentian violet was a messy procedure. Current advances in Canesten and Nystatin formulas have made them more effective, and with the patients becoming more aware of the part they themselves play in causing their own thrush, things generally are beginning to look up. I shall go to town on the patients' preventive role later on.

Cervical Polyps

By the time you get your first diagnosed and treated cervical polyp you may well already know that you are inclined to be a 'polypy' person. Perhaps you have had nasal polyps as a child or teenager. There are several sorts of polyps, including large pendulous things growing singly, or groups of smaller ones looking like the surface of the moon.

They can take ages to develop or they can arrive in a matter of weeks. When the discharge from them is sufficient to maintain a steady liquid drip, bacteria may thrive in it and urinary twinges or full-blooded cystitis will start.

Intercourse can puncture and split the polyps and there may be unusual spots of blood on the sheets. This is another sure sign of any sort of vaginal or cervical growth and should never be ignored. It's there to be helpful, like a signpost.

Go to a good gynaecologist and let him/her have a look.

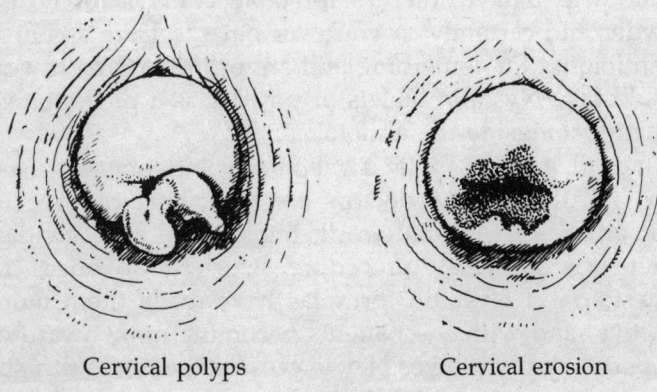

Cervical polyps   Cervical erosion

If he/she says that there is a polyp but 'it seems fairly harmless looking', take a deep breath and say that you would like it off now please, in case the trouble worsens. Say it quite positively and ask how he/she proposes to do this.

Depending upon the polyp, twisting it off or freezing it off with cryosurgery are both simple, quick and pain free. Twisting is pain free but not ache free, for there can be a period-type ache but nothing that two painkillers won't stop. Very occasionally a polyp can be cancerous. The gynaecologist will send the polyp off to the lab – watch him put it in a little sterile bottle and if he doesn't, ask him to do so. I've had polyps in my nose and two on the cervix – no cancer – I'm just polypy!

For three or four days there will be a sloughing of the cervix as the raw patch heals. You don't get scabbing of wounds in such areas – sloughing is what happens instead. It looks just like the end of a period so it probably requires a sanitary pad.

Help your cervix to heal by resting for a couple of days. Don't go jogging or anything, just take time off to sit down on a sofa or up on the bed with a good book, or watch the telly. Sit or lie with your legs apart. Take the weight off the pelvis and you'll recover all the faster. If the polyp had harboured infection, spreading it around the cervix and even contaminating the urine, then a course of appropriate antibiotics would be indicated.

Cervical Erosion

You remember from the last chapter that the cervix has a central canal or tube which leads up into the uterus. This canal can undergo epithelial (skin) changes due to hormone activity in pregnancy, which also enlarges the cervix itself to help it expand enough for birthing. Sometimes the canal epithelium doesn't return to size after birthing and this extra epithelium remains and even continues to grow so that it starts to protrude out of the cervix itself.

Doctors are getting ever lazier about removing erosion, arguing that it's quite a common thing and best left alone. Now this is not the case because each patient knows full well whether it's bothering *her*! Intercourse may hurt, there may be bleeding or a rotten little discharge that stains or itches but may not fit the textbook discharges.

You will have to pluck up the courage – and I do know that it takes courage – to ask politely but firmly for it to be frozen or cauterized away. Should you not have the courage in the face of an obstinate doctor, go elsewhere until someone agrees to your request. Here's a real case for private health insurance.

I have seen so many poor women stumbling around with discharging cervical erosions affecting their daily lives. Don't allow yourself to be abandoned in this way by a doctor. If you've got symptoms and a proven erosion get the treatment for it.

If it's a little erosion it can be frozen off on the couch, but if it's big and the cervical canal is actually blocked by it so that menstrual blood can't get out then an overnight stay in hospital for a general anaesthetic is recommended.

Recovery is as for polyps. There will probably be greater sloughing and you should certainly rest for a week, especially if you have had a general anaesthetic. Don't attempt intercourse for three to four weeks or, better still, wait on for a full monthly cycle until the first menstrual bleed has happened. More sloughing may come away with it. Do remember to go back six weeks later for an all-clear check.

The Wart Virus

This is now becoming very common. If you are sexually active you should regard everything on your hands with suspicious interest, warts included. I happen to have counselled recently a young unmarried couple who have intercourse regularly at weekends when they meet, and on days off or during holidays. The girl is nineteen and a nurse in her final year of training. She was recently put on the children's ward and to her interest contracted a couple of finger warts which she doubtless rubbed or scratched as they were forming.

Out of the blue, she went down with a nasty vaginal discharge and cystitis. She had never had symptoms like this before. She raged at her boyfriend, accusing him of 'giving' something to her and marched off to the hospital gynaecologist who found a nest of warts on the cervix exuding a runny liquid laden with virus.

In lovemaking, her two finger warts could have transmitted the virus to herself or to him first and then into her vagina in foreplay. She had them frozen off the cervix and her fingers but if the virus has penetrated the epithelial cervical or vaginal lining then she may expect further bouts until the virus wanes of its own accord. She could, between contracting it and being treated for it, have transmitted it to her boyfriend. (Incubation for the wart virus *condyloma acuminatum* can vary from one to six months.) That this nineteen-year-old nurse was well until a month after developing her finger warts shows how virulent warts are. Until going on the children's ward where warts are, of course, more prevalent than other wards, she was uninfected.

This is a wonderful illustration of lifestyle and circumstances dictating our bodily condition. Warts are very infectious. Hygiene is all and treatment should be speedy.

Carcinoma of the Cervix

This same girl has a friend, also nineteen, who has cancer of the cervix. She began intercourse at fifteen. *The younger you commence intercourse, the heavier are your chances of having your cervix removed for cancer later on in life.*

Give your body chemistry a chance to grow up fully so that it can repel malignant cells. Get on with sports, hobbies, academic work and travel until you are nineteen-plus. Once you start intercourse you will want more sex, so try hard not to start early. I think that coeducational schools have placed the girls in a dangerous position, for the sexual pressures on them are most unfair. Classwork suffers and so does health.

Cancerous cells of several kinds can grow in the cervical canal or very visibly on the vaginal side of the cervix. You may not know that you have a problem because in its early stages cervical cancer can be symptom free, but as it grows there will be all sorts of symptoms including urinary infection, back ache, discharge, bleeding between periods or after intercourse and pain on intercourse.

Such symptoms will worsen if a gynaecologist doesn't 'find' you in good time. The cancer will spread to include uterus, ovaries, and then onward round the body.

At best you may lose your cervix and the normal means of becoming pregnant. At worst you may die.

Pelvic Infections and the IUD

Almost any heavy bacterial infection of the vagina can rise up through the cervical canal into the uterus and Fallopian tubes. Likewise bacteria from established ovarian cysts can travel down the tubes into the uterus.

Bacteria in large amounts which embed themselves in epithelium (skin) that is weakening under the attack can spread through and around the organs in the pelvis. If infection is in the tubes it is called salpingitis.

If you know that you are prone to vaginal infections and discharges – some of us are and some of us aren't – it is crazy to have any kind of intrauterine device fitted for contraception. Bacteria are not stupid, they will choose the fastest route in their invasion and the string of IUDs will act like a swing bridge over a chasm, straight across instead of trekking around!

Because the aim of the IUD is to keep the cervical canal slightly dilated and prevent a fertilized egg from embedding itself in the uterine wall, there is obviously a larger opening for bacteria to gain entrance to the uterus. If cystitis or discharge or any pain begins with the insertion of an IUD, don't hesitate – have it out straight away.

Those women already scarred both externally and internally by birthing and medical injuries are another huge group who should not contemplate the IUD. Old scars are also welcome routes for marching germs. An IUD may open up an old scar, chafe, or just be an additional hazard.

Discharges start if bacteria get a hold on the string and cystitis will probably follow. Discharges from pelvic infections are profuse also from neisseria gonorrhoea, chlamydia trachomatis and anaerobic bacteriodes or cocci. With E. Coli or streptococcus coming from the bowels of the sufferer herself you will realize that even pelvic infections can in some way be self-caused. It can be possible to have a contaminated water supply from the taps themselves or in the cistern but ninety-nine point nine per cent of these pelvic infections are initially self-sown.

You need plenty of antibiotics for pelvic infections, so plenty of Nystatin oral tablets if you're thrush prone, plenty of fluids, plenty of mineral and vitamin supplements, plenty of effective hygiene and plenty of rest. All bacteria spread faster if you walk round – don't.

Sit or lie down during the treatments and for God's sake don't have intercourse. You'll feel too ill anyway!

Normal Discharges

Each woman has her own level of daily vaginal secretion. It can vary according to the time of the month, whether she is on the Pill, pregnant, having intercourse regularly or not having it regularly.

The older you get the drier you get generally. If you have recently had a discharge, the vaginal epithelium may not have recovered its natural flow and the pH balance may still be upset, so attempts at intercourse will need KY jelly and some care.

The discharge that most sexually active women, or women on the Pill for reasons other than contraception, have is a thick white mucous. It varies in amount, but can be heavy enough to ooze out of the vagina and make the perineum too sticky for comfort. It can be contained by hygiene so that on its worst days removal of the overnight collection when you get up will keep you comfortable until the evening when the day collection can be removed.

After passing urine stay on the loo and pour a bottle of cool water down the perineum, stick the third or large finger of the hand which is not holding the bottle up the vagina as far as the cervix, and hook out the discharge until your finger is coming out much clearer. Dry the perineum completely with a towel and you will find the days become much more comfortable. Don't use a bidet ever. *Understanding Cystitis* explains the hazards fully.

The discharge in pregnancy is so rich in hormones that you may find it quite irritative. Ask for swabs if you are worried, but if hygiene is good the chances of negative bacterial results are also good. Just keep washing the discharge out with water (no soap) and clean, scrubbed fingers.

Whether you have a very heavy discharge, a burning dry vagina or variations in between, you must seek the help of a competent gynaecologist. Discharges and vaginal conditions are so quick to influence the bladder that examination and appropriate treatment can be necessary within forty-eight hours of the trouble becoming obvious.

I have mostly found it essential to have access to several medical personnel. I have my own private health insurance, two general practitioners, one National Health and one private, two gynaecologists, and access to the special clinic in a teaching hospital. I rarely see any of them, but in the past years of suffering, such access has helped enormously to deal correctly and swiftly with my highly-sensitive skin, bad childbirth and cystitis.

The hallmark, I have found, of a good woman's doctor is the presence of a microscope in the consulting room, plus a shelf of sterile tubes and bottles for full laboratory sample analysis. After that the doctor must be prepared to listen to the circumstances surrounding the current trouble and talk as much about self-help as prescribable treatment. One also feels much more at ease with the gynaecologist who isn't rushed, who has warm hands and who begins the physical examination in what is called the dorsal position (flat on your back). This is the position most normal and relaxing for a woman. It is not pleasant to go straight into a left lateral (side) and expose the anal opening. The speculum, which is used to prop open the vaginal walls, should be warm and inserted first, if possible, before fingers, so as not to re-arrange the mucous needed for cytological smears. Your breathing is nervous at this point and you should help the gynaecologist by keeping your arms at your side – the instinct is to put them behind your head – and taking good, if forced, breath to try to relax the abdominal muscles. If they are very tense, and the vagina too, the gynaecologist will have his/her work cut out to examine you thoroughly.

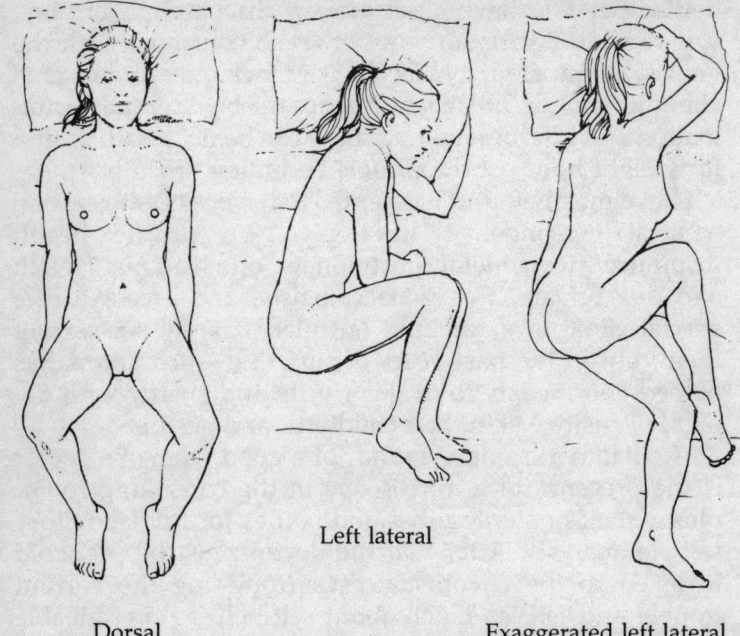

Left lateral

Dorsal   Exaggerated left lateral

Gynaecological examination

Of course, if you know and trust the gynaecologist well because he/she is the regular one who is gentle, then examination is less of a tense affair. The beauty of having a private health insurance is that you can go on until you do find a nice one who uses common sense in conjunction with great expertise. The State gynaecologists are often chancily varied and seeing the same one twice is uncommon. They just don't realize how nice it is for us to see a familiar face!

Why many women never see a gynaecologist from one year to the next mystifies me. Women come to me for counselling and when I get to the appropriate point in note-taking I'm astounded at the numbers who haven't been gynaecologically examined in three or more years, yet some silly doctor has been packing them with antibiotics or has missed some vital gynaecological symptom like back ache and done absolutely nothing about referring to an expert. *If you have a vagina you must use gynaecologists.* If your vagina is sexually active it needs *more* attention not less.

Bacteria and their Origins

There are many unusual bacteria that can find their way up the vagina to the cervix. The VD or special clinic may not mention such bacteria if they are not sexually transmittable, nor may it comment upon other sorts of cervical irregularities.

Here are some bacteria and their origin.

Klebsiella A group with several strains but most usually waterborne as external contamination, or from swallowing bad water.

Pseudomonas Aeruginosa (frequently found in hospital departments).

Neisseria Pharyngis, Catarrhalis (both possible from oral sex), Gonorrhoea.

Proteus Mirabilis, Vulgaris (enjoy an alkaline medium. Also found in renal pelvic condition and septicaemia).

Streptococci Faecalis (from bowels), Haemolytic (from skin infections), Pyogenes (from nose and throat), Pneumoniae (from lungs).

E. Coli (Escherichia coliform) Faecal serotypes are 01, 02, 04, 06, 07, 025, 050 (from the small intestines and bowels).

Staphylococcus Aureus (found in the lower respiratory tract), Epidermitis, Saprophyhcus, Albus (from bladder catheterization).

Yeasts (Candida/monilia) Albicans, Stellatoidea, Tropicalis, Krusei, Pseudo Tropicalis, Parapsilosis, Guilliermondii, Norvegensis.

Rhodoturula Rubra.

Trichomonas Vaginalis Mycoplasma Hominis, Toralopsis Glabrata, Castellii, Inconspicua, Holmii, Saccharomyces Cervisae.

Haemophilus Inluenzae Parainfluenzae, Vaginalis, Ducreyi (soft chancroid).

Chlamydia Trachomatis Chlamydia B. (a type frequently found in birds and can be passed to people in contact with domestic/wild birds).

Gardnerella Vaginalis Otherwise known as Corynebacterium Vaginale or H. Vaginalis (thin discharge).

In 1966 Gordan et al showed the frequency of occurrence of various organisms in *normal* vaginal flora, taken from a sample of women.

Haemophilus Vaginalis	9.8
Corynebacterium (diptheroids)	39.0
Mycoplasma (PPLO)	15.3
Lactobacilli (Doderlein)	81.0
Coliform	12.2
Aerobic Streptococci	24.2
Strep Faecalis	0.0
Anaerobic organisms	21.0
Staph Aureus	0.0
Candida	9.7

Prevention

If you have any of the diseases or discharges that I've mentioned, or others of your own particular home-grown variety, then you will certainly want to know what you can do about them. Prevention of such disasters or discomforts is miles better than the agonies of mind and body when yet another attack looks imminent.

Why not take simple daily care of the vagina and perineum just as you would your teeth, face and hair?

In the sixth and vastly updated edition of Sir John Peel's and J H. Brudenell's *Textbook of Gynaecology*, the two men stress the need to revise their work on gynaecological disorders because of changing social and psychological factors. They add new chapters on cytology, family planning and sexual problems which now play such an important part in modern gynaecology. And all this was way back in 1969! They also say quite clearly that: 'Because of its proximity to the genital organs, the bladder is often involved in gynaecological disorders.' Read that again reinterpreted by me as, 'Gynaecological disorders are often associated with bladder disorders.'

This update was published during my own private hell of cystitis and discharges from 1966–71, and in their textbook are the clear directions for 'scrupulous hygiene' that I thought I was discovering and pioneering!

What do today's practising gynaecologists, urologists and family doctors read in medical school? Do they take any notice of common sense and logic when diagnosing a patient with vaginal diseases? Perhaps they leave such matters to the platform of medical writers like me who are not practising medicine but who nevertheless are informed and have opinions.

There is no doubt that my early and subsequent work on cystitis and associated conditions has broken new ground not only for sufferers but also for many top specialists who applaud such clear spelling out of common sense and simple preventative directives for their own use in the training school or consulting room.

So here now is a solid section of prevention of the diseases we have just looked at.

Trichomonas

1 Put a sheet of loo paper in the pan to stop faecal back-splash in a deep lavatory pan before passing a stool. Lavatory water contains Trichomonas.

2 If the lavatory has an unusually shallow pan and you need to flush it at an intermediate stage, get up and wait for the flushing water to subside. Don't flush yourself, too!

3 Wash your hands with soap and hot water after using toilet paper.

4 Re-soap one hand and with that hand soap the anal orifice only, nothing else, until it's bubbly. A pure soap, not perfumed, coloured antiseptic or deodorized is recommended.

5 Rinse that hand very well under running warm water and then scrub under the nails of it with a nailbrush.

6 Fill up any medium-sized mineral water bottle – not a milk bottle or carton – with *warm* water. It must be warm because faecal material from the bowels is greasy and won't wash off with cool water. Obviously hot water must not be used because the skin is too tender. If you are out of your own bathroom and you forgot to take your bottle, acquire one from somewhere, the very, very last resort is the bathroom mug. Wash it out well and use several fill-ups to do the same job as the bottle, which is:

7 Sit back on the lavatory, pointing your back passage, as the lowest part of your bottom, down the loo. Pour the warm water down the labia, vulva and perineum and with the spare hand clean around the inner labia, up into the vagina and finally ensure that all the soap is off the anus. If the vagina seems mucky fill up the bottle again and hook out as much mucous as you can. Ensure all soapy bubbles are gone from the anus.

8 Pat the vulva and perineum thoroughly dry with a guest towel or face cloth that is only kept for this purpose and changed once a week.

If you pass wind a lot for whatsoever reason, or if your bowels only move every two or more days, this simple bottle washing must be done once a day anyway as a freshener. I have myself, only very recently, had a mild E. Coli urinary infection, the first since the early 1970s because I had intercourse on a vulva that had not been fully bottle washed as above, for thirty-nine hours. I hadn't passed a stool in that time so I hadn't washed. I had poured cool water over it but that alone is insufficient to counteract wind-borne E. Coli.

Candida Albicans (also called thrush, monilia or yeast).

You can buy books on this subject but following the logic of the body you will restrict upsurges of this fungus that is always present in the gut in small, unsymptomatic levels by:

1 Removing glucose and sugar from your diet because candida lives on it.

2 Removing as much man-refined carbohydrate food from your diet as possible because it converts to sugar in the body.

The starch from white flour converts in the body to glucose, and refined sugar – which is concentrated amounts of sugar processed from sugar beet and cane – also converts to glucose. These two main carbohydrates are the prime sources of excessive glucose circulating in the bloodstream that serve to fuel the growth of candida. Glucose, except in diabetes, is not found in urine but it is expelled, as we have previously read, by our lungs in carbon dioxide when we breathe out.

I recommend a careful reading of *The Saccharine Disease* by T.C. Cleave, now deceased, who spent a lifetime working on carbohydrate intake and whose work pioneered carbohydrate-related diseases.

A look at the carbohydrate table in the Appendix (page 204) will give you a rough idea of what to avoid, rotate or reduce in your diet, if you want to take thrush seriously. It's the refined ones that are worst not the fresh foods. Refined foods per relative twelve grams are four or five times more loaded with sugar than the fresh foods which are heavier in bulk weight. Potatoes and rice are unexpectedly high carriers of carbohydrate – watch out!

3 It has also been reported that whilst the taking of the Pill does not directly cause thrush it may impair the metabolic rate of carbohydrate assimilation and breakdown so encouraging mild levels of steroid diabetes. There is no doubt in practice that Pill-users are a big group of thrush sufferers, so if thrush starts and arises frequently whilst you are on the Pill you must contemplate coming off it.

4 The relationship between antibiotics and thrush is well known and I recommend Nystatin oral tablets or powder to be taken every time you need a course of antibiotics, as a preventative.

5 The vaginal acid/alkaline balance is also important. Thrush grows in an alkaline environment – the bloodstream is alkaline – so is the vagina for a few days before a period. At such a time insert a lactic acid pessary high up to the cervix once a day for those few days to regain acidity.

6 Since alkaline blood passes down the vagina during a period, some people may get thrush after a period. On the sixth or seventh day of bleeding, wash out the vagina with a bottle of cool water and insert a lactic

acid pessary for three or four days to restore acidity and deprive thrush of alkalinity.

Lactic acid pessaries are available without prescription at most pharmacies. A manufacturer is Richard Daniel and Son Ltd of Derby, England, Ortho-Cilag Pharmaceuticals Ltd of High Wycombe, Bucks, England make Aci-Jel therapeutic vaginal jelly which has a similar action but some women can experience a slight stinging from it. Again it can be bought without prescription.

Lactic acid pessaries are more sophisticated than natural yoghurt which is very messy and smacks of street corner feminism. Any dose of candida can only be helped by lactic acid but it should not be seen as a major vaginal preventative for candida except in the before-listed circumstances – full knowledgeable prevention is the main aim.

All of the following points are extremely important:

- Eat three or four tablespoons of live yoghurt before any meal to line the stomach with lactobacilli.
- Don't eat sweets or chocolates.
- Don't drink alcohol, canned sodas or juices. Alcohol converts to sugar.
- Avoid cheeses and other yeast/fermenting foods.
- Two baths or showers only each week, not too hot. Get in, wash, get out. Thrush likes warmth and moisture – a bath is just that.
- Swimming in treated water has an antiseptic action on the perineal skin and inside the vagina. It will promote the growth of yeast.
- Wearing lycra/nylon clothing such as leotards for keep fit, jogging, dancing and so on heightens body heat and sweating. Thrush loves a hot body.
- Sunbathing in a lycra/nylon suit promotes thrush both

from the sun's heat by the trapping of perineal perspiration.

- Sexual intercourse can ping-pong thrush. It is sexually transmittable. The friction in intercourse again promotes a higher vaginal temperature, and body temperature. Use a sheath but better still don't have intercourse until a clearance check. Cool the vagina after sex with a bottle of cold water.
- Jeans cause perineal perspiration. Jean seams add clitoral and urethral bruising. Throw them away.
- Any restrictive outer clothing like trousers or tailored skirts prevents cooling air from drying the vulva. Wear looser clothing.
- Tights and nylon panties also cause sweating and stop air. Only wear stockings, suspender belts and cotton panties.
- Go without underwear whenever possible. Slips or petticoats are fine.
- Don't sit all day on the edge of the office chair. Allow the vulva to breathe and dry out.
- Cut pubic hair to half an inch every four or five weeks at the same time as you do toenails, because pubic hair retains perineal sweat and the enlarged hair follicles trap fungus.
- Bedding should be warm but 'breathing'. Use cotton sheets and blankets if you share a double bed. Terylene duvets will increase sweating though down duvets may be all right.
- Wear cotton nighties – not pyjamas and certainly no undies in bed.

Having said all that, large numbers of women have 'deeper' thrush, thrush that sits in the gut in a permanent 'overload' situation. After all the antibiotics that I ate in the late 'sixties and early 'seventies for my cystitis, my gut has remained in 'overload' with this miserable fungus.

There's no doubt that I can control about eighty per cent of that overload by restraint and with great care, but I do benefit from additional help.

Three times a year I am desensitized to candida (along with other allergies). In order for these desensitizing injections to work I prepare for ten days beforehand. If I don't, then the injection doesn't work properly. In those ten days I stop all alcohol and lower all carbohydrate and sugar intake. I also take Nystatin oral powder in water three or four times each day (tablets might do instead). This effort brings down my overload gut candida and allows the injection to act like gelatin and 'set' the gut level at this low point. In the months that follow, I have no obvious candida and it's absolute bliss to have a cheese sandwich and a lager!

This year I learnt some more about thrush. For years I have written the sentence 'thrush will arise if you are debilitated'. I thought I understood this but a sequence of events has really hammered it home to me. 1987 was a very grim year for me. I have had to contend with much personal trouble and mountains of stress which finally required professional help. A period in this year also involved helping an eighty-four-year-old great aunt through distressing terminal illnesses and on into reluctantly accepting death.

My sleep patterns went and sleep itself simply wasn't refreshing me. I fought it – refusing sleeping pills – and walked round in permanent misery and crawling tiredness. Then throat infections and an injured arm added to everything else. Thrush kept me company all year and I had some really bad episodes which put me in bed as I couldn't even walk because of it. Finally I gave in to the sleeping pills and took over three weeks to resume some normality and make up the lost hours' sleep. As this got better and I slept, so thrush calmed down as well. It was a dramatic pointer to the rightness of the old adage about debilitation and made me fully aware of its meaning. I don't wait for crawling tiredness before taking action and I take greater care now in view of advancing menopause not to overstretch my body's resources.

The other fascination at this awful time was my great aunt's final ten days in a hospice. I've never watched dying on a daily basis before. She took no food, only sips of liquid which caused instant vomiting and, therefore, all pills were stopped. On her bedside locker appeared one day oral Nystatin drops for her tongue. The wind coming out of every orifice was due to a complete takeover of her body by candida. Every part of her was going down to fungus invasion. If her tongue was an indication of events in the rest of her body, then amazing things were going on.

I learnt a lot about debilitation. All sorts of things can cause tiredness. Acute or chronic tiredness must be stopped and life revised. Make a list of things which cause tiredness. It could be several pages long and may include: pain, menopause, too much sexual activity, giving birth, breast-feeding, all kinds of stress, dieting, poor sleep, being up too late, looking after dependants, divorce, rows, long shopping trips, Christmas, too much housework, the wrong job, travelling to and from work, work itself and so on. Have a good think.

Sleeping pills are only a temporary aid. Don't get hooked. Use them sparingly, but don't wait as long as I did!

That we have this combination of self-help and medical help for thrush is due to an immense increase in thrush over the past twenty-five years. Modern life is entirely responsible and information must be relayed to sufferers and doctors. Thrush is preventable.

Wart Virus and Herpes

As with all sexually transmittable diseases, you should be absolutely honest before having intercourse with a stranger about the presence of a discharge, or warts, herpes, chlamydia, thrush, syphilis, gonorrhoea, pubic lice (crabs), worms, Aids, and scabies.

The sheath is the only barrier. Carry it in a wallet and use it. The vagina and penis will then have some protection. Any viral upsurge as with herpes should make you forgo sex for the three or four-week period of its presence.

Anyone with a lip sore should be avoided like the plague. No kissing, no touching and put restrictions on towels, serviettes, crockery, cutlery, with those items being separately washed away from others in the home. Sadly, the Communion cup now becomes suspicious.

Warts on the hands or any hand contact with warty genitalia should be regarded as contagious. Hot water, antiseptic, antiseptic soap and a scrubbing brush should be employed on the hands at the first opportunity and thereafter. Go for a vaginal and cervical swab to check out possible transference of the hand infection internally. Warts internally and externally can and should be cauterized or frozen. If you work with, or have children who grow a wart, treatment must be sought in case someone sexually active has skin contact with them.

Cervical Erosion

As I said previously, this will drip and its only treatment is to seek medical help. However, if you know how to clean out the vagina you can restrain and restrict the drip a little bit and be more comfortable.

Use the bottle-washing method (as described in *Trichomonas*) scrupulously to remove invasive bowel-perineal bacteria as much as possible. Then refill the bottle and, sitting back on the lavatory once more, tilt your buttocks

87

and pelvis to get really good access of the finger into the vagina. Pour the water slowly into the cupped palm of the hand whose finger is inside. As that finger pulls and hooks there will be room for the water to get inside too. Keep at it with the finger and water for a minute and the resulting cleaning will stop the cervical drip from causing soreness and inflammation on the vulva for a few hours.

Pelvic Infections

Again hygiene, as per the bottle washing, will prevent all rising infections from the perineum. As I have said, that is the commonest route for such infections so take the daily bottle washing with great seriousness – it is protecting all the pelvic organs both renal and productive.

Normal Discharges

There is volume and colour variation throughout the monthly cycle, but if at any time this non-bacterial discharge (do get it checked if it is too heavy) causes slight irritation, uncomfortable wetness or soreness then wash it out just as previously discussed. You will be bottle washing after a bowel movement anyway, so that's the usual time to clean out the vagina, but a freshener at night-time is nice and, as you'll see later, is incorporated into pre- and post-intercourse routines.

If Sir John Peel, the Queen's past gynaecologist and myself are both in favour of absolutely 'scrupulous hygiene', you can bet it's the right thing to do! So please work away at the proper perineal hygiene taught here. Don't use a bidet, squat in the bath, sit over the sink or any other manner of procedure. You must do the bottle washing absolutely precisely as I have described.

E.Coli Cystitis

All adult women, and also children with bacteria in their urine samples, should wash precisely as tabled under

Trichomonas (page 80). But I cannot tell you how important it is to wash in this way every day. I say 'every day' because of a new situation I personally faced very recently. I always wash without fail as described every time I pass a stool and I always freshen up quickly an hour or so before intercourse is likely. On this occasion, I had passed a stool on *Tuesday* morning and done the full soap/bottle washing as usual. Late on *Wednesday* afternoon I had intercourse, not having passed a stool during Wednesday. I had freshened up with a bottle of coolish tap water before getting into bed, but no full soap routine because I hadn't passed a stool and didn't think I needed to wash.

Twenty-four hours later,I began twingeing and it wasn't soreness, it felt decidedly more ominous. I instigated a good urine test, and sure enough there was a mild E. Coli count. I needed Erithromycin antibiotics, so the sensitivity culture dictated, and on pondering how I could have allowed E. Coli to stray, I concluded it was a natural 'leakage' not aborted by hygiene because of the thirty-hour interval between the last full bottle washing and 'freshener' before intercourse. So do wash fully each and every day, more especially if you are sexually active.

E. Coli cystitis is the commonest cause of sexual cystitis. Stray bowel bacteria is rubbed forwards in manual and penile intercourse, so that it might invade the urethra. Once there, it will rise quickly into the bladder and cause distressing cystitis.

Contraceptives

Assuming the perineum, vagina, vulva, bladder etc. are all well and capable of having intercourse, it is then essential to decide if the end result of intercourse, i.e. a baby, is wanted. It is my belief that a child needs both a mother and a father; childhood is best enjoyed when there are at least two adults participating in the rearing process. Children need a protected environment whilst they become acquainted with risks, dangers and traditional behaviour. Such an environment will help to encourage health and welfare and diminish stress on one parent.

The strain of such constancy on one parent, may lead to poor loving and loss of later companionship, so I believe that until proper back-up provision exists in the life of the mother, on whom most of the constancy depends anyway, conception is best avoided. Contraception still largely falls on the woman, especially since the western nations thought that all problems were solved with the discovery of the Pill.

After this, men abandoned the sheath and revelled in the new-found sensations and feels of the freed penis. Women relaxed away from the fear of pregnancy and also enjoyed the delight of skin to skin contact with an uninterrupted ejaculation and climax. Contraception in modernized countries had really only been abstinence, withdrawal, then condoms, the diaphragm (Dutch cap) and the Pill. That intercourse could now take place with complete protection against pregnancy and without any messy vaginal or penile preparation, was tremendously exciting for both sexes.

Manufacturers, spurred by thoughts of profit, newly available medical knowledge and engineering processes began to devise and test other methods of contraception. Spermicidal creams, foams, and pessaries were marketed and made non-prescribable so that any woman could have effective contraception instantly.

The coil was offered in the late 1960s as a new fool-proof method for those unable to tolerate the Pill. It had the major disadvantage of necessitating medical fitment and that successful fitment was dependent upon the doctor's skill – occasionally lacking. Again, drawbacks slowly surfaced.

The 'morning after' injection of heavy doses of hormones and the new cervical sponges of spermicidal agents are more recent additions to the market.

One thing has been learned in the last forty years. It is that not all contraceptives may suit every patient. If I were to map out the contraceptive requirements and practices of any female in an idealistic way it would be:

1 Abstinence until nineteen to twenty-one years old to lessen risks of cervical illnesses.
2 The sheath until a strong regular relationship developed.
3 Six months of any year on a low dose Pill and six months of sheath and sponge combinations.
4 If the first six months of the Pill provided any side effects, give it up for good.
5 Perhaps an experimental time with the coil after careful discussion with a good gynaecologist and all relevant individual assessments made.

6 The vaginal sponge, and sheath.
7 Careful cool water douching or the washing out of the vagina in older age.

Now, I fully realise that thousands of doctors and sexually active people would find disagreements, provisos and extra recommendations, and I would in any individual situation be in total agreement. There is no hard and fast way of recommending contraception. It has to be individual, and that individual's life has to start going by so that knowledge of that body is charted. Who knows the foibles of each body and its reactions until it has indeed been given a set of conditions to which to react?

Being now in my mid-forties I am in a good position to view, with hindsight, which contraceptives have suited my body and which have not. Perhaps the reader might find it of interest, remembering that I knew nothing when I began. Living at home until I was twenty-two gave virtually no opportunity for sex at all. Certainly I never slept with anyone so I paid no heed at all to sexual responsibility. Behaviour codes were stronger than they are now for both sexes and you simply got on with having other sorts of good times.

However, from my engagement on, 'heavy petting' became insufficient as nature urged on the mating, and every few weeks of our eight-month engagement an opportunity for being alone would be used. The sheath was an occasional protection, but mostly withdrawal. There was no cystitis or discomfort of any sort, which I now put down to going to the loo and passing urine because we'd be journeying back to base or parental homes and one would naturally clean up before a journey. Doubtless, I would also have wished to have a clean up for fear of anyone guessing what I'd been up to! So maybe I bathed quickly after passing urine. My vagina also had plenty of time to recover – weeks!

From the marriage night on, though, I didn't have to leave my new husband's side so, without having been told the importance of cleaning up, I didn't. I slept in the 'rosy afterglow'. Additionally, my doctor had suggested the vaginal foam Emko as a contraceptive since I had a major abdominal operation in my early twenties. I used Emko for three years without linking the stinging to it. With nasty bouts of cystitis, lovemaking in between and unlinked as a cause, I was frantic to make up for the two or three weeks lost in the cystitis attacks. These sexual bouts would have been leaving a swollen, raw and still small vagina very open to chemical contamination with additional inflammation from the foam contraceptive and sexual thrusting.

A three-week spell on the Pill, a high oestrogen Pill, in 1968, put on a stone in weight and left me dizzy and tearful. My body took six months to recover from it so I steered clear of the Pill for years.

As I now had cystitis very frequently and then also became pregnant, ending with a Caesarian section and long convalescence, there was so little sex that contraception was unnecessary. Withdrawal, Emko and the sheath were used when required. Thrush from all the antibiotics caused such a sore and unhealthy vagina that that also prohibited sex.

When mini-Pills were invented I had a couple of sessions of Minovlar before and after the birth of my son in 1974 with some better success that the earlier brush with the higher dose Pill. But then my husband went abroad in 1975 and this began eight years of partings and irregular sex between us, so I had no need of daily contraception.

Apart from wishing time and again for a less sensitive metabolism, I have, in hindsight, come off lightly in terms of any permanent reaction or damage from man-made contraceptives. I have actively avoided the diaphragm, the coil and sterilization. This stems mostly from that early abdominal operation when my GP and I both felt that there was enough scarring and damaged tissue around the pelvis to put off any extra aggravation.

The Caesarian section of my daughter in 1969 and the inverted uterus (I pushed that out, too, after my son!) in 1974 meant that any foreign bodies were best left well alone, so thankfully all subsequent doctors have excluded the cap and coil as acceptable contraceptives for me. Two gynaecologists repositioned the runaway uterus and it still functions!

Having said to my then husband that I'd had more than enough female trouble and operations for one woman, I now expected him to take over permanent contraceptive responsibility. In 1979 I bought him a vasectomy for Christmas and thus ended some of my own contraceptive headaches.

However, my marriage broke up, so this was not to be the end of my contraceptive responsibility. Sexual intercourse in the two or three years before and after the divorce has varied from roughly six to twenty-five times in any year, and I wasn't prepared to take the Pill when there was no frequent or regular pattern. Thus I cast around and decided on Rendells pessaries, a non-prescribable vaginal tablet, reasonably priced. As a well-taught consumer I obeyed the packet's instructions and inserted a tablet high up to the cervix before penetration. On several occasions I was beset with dreadful soreness and urinary reactions after intercourse. With my knowledge, both of cystitis and my own sensitivities, it was plain as day that I was reacting to the chemicals in the tablets, just as I obviously had with the Emko years earlier.

The packet also relayed the information that the tablet must be in place some minutes before actual ejaculation. But I knew my partner's habits in bed and with his co-operation a moment would arrive when the need for the tablet could be judged. So penile rubbing together with the chemical reaction was minimized by inserting the tablet three minutes before ejaculation. A good wash out afterwards helped to clear the chemicals and sexual secretions away leaving a basically clean vagina and a complete avoidance of reaction for which I was mightily thankful.

This may not be advisable for everyone of course, but neither I nor my partner are heavily fertile, he being in his late fifties and I mid-forties, so I felt the risk of preg-nancy to be not so high.

As it happens, this man is also not regularly available and on a long six-month parting, I became briefly involved with a younger man in his 30s. This, I felt, might demand a return to the low dose Pill but after two months I was riddled with thrush and came off it. The new vaginal sponge 'Today' was being promoted and I decided to research it. I felt its only drawback was its expense, but as an irregularly used, non-prescribable contraceptive giving high protection against contraception, both I and my younger partner liked it. Neither of us had skin reactions and neither felt it impeded enjoyment. The additional complication with this younger man was that he was a 'leaker'. I had never before heard this expression because no man I'd been involved with, as far as I was aware, did this. With an untimeable ejaculation, the sponge had to be placed over the cervix before bedtime and was therefore able to account for the discrepancies and give complete protection throughout penetration.

Finishing off this brief look at my own contraceptive history, I have not used any contraceptives for ten months now. During this time I have had intercourse about ten times with my older partner only. I have adopted the cool water douche method (see page 155) within minutes of intercourse ending. Intercourse has taken place regardless of ovulation times and I, with money in the bank for

95

termination if necessary, am now interested in finding out if I'm fertile or not. I shall still douche as a part protection. Sperm is killed in cool or cold water, but if that's all I now need to do, its a hundred per cent better than suffering any man-made contraceptive reactions. Perhaps I haven't been truly fertile since my inverted uterus in 1974 or perhaps it's my partner's low sperm count. I'd love to know, but even I am not that active a researcher to undergo tests on myself and ask him to as well!

All of this having been said, with much personal sadness, I should add that I have been as careful and hygienic as possible but wish that life itself had been kinder. I would strongly exhort men in particular to pay attention to their general and sexual duties and responsibilities to their female partner. I start with them because statistics show that more women divorce men than vice-versa. Women generally are by nature the more responsible and faithful of the two sexes and do wish to be. Men tend to be the roamers and generally less stable. However, there can be exceptions, and I apply the same exhortations to those of my own sex who take responsibilities too lightly.

On a very recent note, I should remind everyone that because of sexual irresponsibility and travel, the deathly disease of Aids demands at least the use of the sheath. Although I suspect that, as carriers go about their daily lives, with transmission of the virus possible on levels other than sexual intercourse, the sheath will not wholly restrict the world-wide threat to all our lives.

As with suitability of contraceptives for any individual woman, so the diseases and reactions are individually variable. I have met countless women in my adult social life and, of course, in my work with cystitis. There are women who start the Pill in their teens and have happily stayed on it all their sexual lives. Often such women may go into a decline when they finally stop taking it! I'm not one for medical scare stories, but I respect the thoughts of those who get frightened. Many healthy women have needlessly come off the Pill in a scare only to find a reaction to the contraceptive with which it has been replaced.

Others have mild reactions when they started on the Pill and fail to experiment with another type, so denying themselves some years of worry-free intercourse. And all of us have met women who have nasty reactions to all brands. The key to successful Pill-taking is a really good gynaecologist who will stick with you as you experiment in your search for the most suitable brand.

The IUD is less popular, probably because if trouble starts, you yourself can't do anything about it, only a doctor can. The coil needs insertion and removal by a doctor so appointments have to be made, which means delays. The coil is also a very visible piece of rather unattractive engineering and many women feel a bit shuddery at the idea of that thing sitting inside them. It hasn't a trouble-free history, either. It can get lost and the string can encourage vaginal infections. Nasty pelvic inflammatory diseases can be traced to insertion of a coil, and if the doctor inserting it damages even minutely any part of the structure, then damage can also result to the uterine wall.

It always strikes me as odd that men try not to be made to use the sheath because they don't like putting it on, yet so many men and male doctors fail to understand that women might not enjoy preparing female contraception! How would men get on if they had to put their legs in stirrups for a coil insertion and then live daily as it settles down in their system with, for instance, heavy bleeding or back ache. How would men get on if they had to have sheaths custom-made and fitted as the cap must be, and then have the great joy of sizing up the possibility of intercourse happening, shoving this large rubber dome with rigid edges up themselves having squirted a spermicidal jelly all round it? Then, after sex, feeling up themselves and pulling the whole mucky mess back down again, washing the rubber cap and putting it away in a box until next time?

No man I can think of would put up with all that and have the grace to be a good lover!

It may well be that the current generation of forty and fifty year old men are better lovers than younger men because in the 1950s and 1960s withdrawal of the penis just before ejaculation made for a bit more planning and design. So did calculating the point at which the sheath should be put on. Both ways made for lengthier and cleverer sexual prowess to forestall climax. However, once the Pill emerged as an unseen and effective contraceptive, young men could ejaculate immediately and stay inside all the time. We've always heard that older men are often better lovers, taking more time to serve and please and exercising better ejaculatory control, but how much of that is just due to older age and experience? Could some of it be due to early contraceptive practices? If so, are we about to lose those skilled men of their generations? It's a thought. I shall be talking about the art and skills of making love later on because if it *is* skilled it adds enormously to the likelihood of pain free and reaction free intercourse for the woman.

All contraceptives are capable of causing urethritis and cystitis. All contraceptives are capable of causing vaginal, cervical and uterine disorders. All contraceptives should, therefore, be thoughtfully used by everyone.

Anytime that you have intercourse and can, with the help of this book, relate trouble down below to that intercourse, it could be worthwhile checking out your contraceptive amongst other things.

Recap

So you're about to have intercourse and you have made many thoughtful background preparations:

- A healthy set of reproductive organs.
- A healthy set of renal organs.
- A disease-free body.
- An emptied bowel and bladder.
- Clean teeth – (its nicer!).
- A tube of lubricating jelly near by.
- An aroused man!
- A cleaned perineum and properly bottle-washed anus.
- A well lubricated vagina.
- A well washed penis!
- An appropriate contraceptive.
- Clean and smooth fingernails (him too!).
- Not too much acid alcohol circulating in the bloodstream!

PART TWO

Having Intercourse

Foreplay

Sexual Cystitis is not a sexy book. At least, I don't intend it to be so. What the individual reader feels is not due to any overt descriptive phraseology on my part. I only want people in health or self-help difficulties to be able to overcome them and have the choice of having a straightforward, enjoyable sex life. I feel strongly about it because I don't feel I have had a straightforward and regular sex life myself.

There were a lot of things about sex that I didn't know which undoubtedly would have helped my ex-husband and me to 'bond' in our early years of marriage. My honeymoon and the first five years of marriage were a sexual nightmare which, in the light of later knowledge, was totally and utterly unnecessary because of bladder and vaginal illness unwittingly self-caused.

It is that unnecessary aspect that fills me with fury and tearful sadness. But to blame myself totally is unrealistic. I obviously have and had then a sensitive skin, although it can't be that sensitive since the self-help learned and employed over the years has been a hundred per cent successful: no cystitis proper since 1971 and only three attacks since then, all absolutely accounted for in special circumstances.

My mother never told me a thing about preparation for

sex, but then presumably she had never needed to know for herself because to my knowledge she's only ever had one dose of mild cystitis – when she was in her sixties. I've never known her visit a gynaecologist except for treatment for a miscarriage when I was eleven, and I don't to this day know whether she ever washed before and after intercourse. She had never experienced sexual illness or cystitis at all, let alone to the horrific extent that I had by the time I was just twenty-five years old. There were no sisters to chat to, no regular job with girls' talk, no magazine or media items and no books on sexual preparation or health.

I mention this again to let you, the reader, know that I fully sympathize with and comprehend your own frustrations and furies if your sex life is an uninterrupted misery.

From a position of choice, people only want intercourse with someone who is nice to them. Someone who has not created any sort of suffering, someone who shows a loving and caring disposition to them. Choice can come shaded, but overall your bedroom mate is, or should be, to your liking – your choice.

Of course, it's also your choice to be celibate, or to say no.

It is not always your choice to be without a sexual partner at all – that comes under the general heading of life – but when you are actually in the bedroom, you do both choose one another for participation in the act of intercourse.

The average woman still 'waits' for the man to approach her. I mean to say, generally speaking, that it's not the woman who walks across a room and asks a man out to a meal! 'Can I see you again?' is still said mainly by men. So, in its ultimate conclusion, the woman doesn't know whether that man will be a good sexual partner until intercourse has happened a few times. And, of course, he himself doesn't know whether he had excellent, average or poor ratings as a lovemaker because he doesn't have lessons from, or the viewpoints of, other males making love. He can read porn and watch blue movies all night, but if he has no inner sense of rhythm, timing or excitement within his own mind he won't be able to transfer those skills into his hands, hips, and loins.

Women are cheerful and encouraging in the main during lovemaking with a chosen partner. If he's not that brill, so what? At least you are having intercourse and enjoying some parts of it. It takes a very extrovert and brave woman to tell a man how to perform in a new position if he has never himself suggested it and if he's not too good at it, or even to tell him he's no good at all!

The nearest equation to this, perhaps, can be thought of in a dance-floor situation. If *every* man in the room can technically do the waltz, invariably some will be more rhythmic, more demanding, more aggressive in guiding you. They will also vary in height and width, lightness of foot and firmness of hand in the small of your back. Skills in bed are no different.

Torvill and Dean, those fabulous skaters, held the world in ecstasy as they responded to one another's skills and undoubted sexual expression. The 'match' of male and female – not just the 'chase' – is tirelessly rewarding and is the ultimate aim of dating. Jayne Torvill matches Christopher Dean with her superb interpretations of feminity and responsiveness to his strong masculine lead. It is just as important in sexual intercourse for the woman to respond to whatever is being implemented as it is for the man to respond to anything she feels like doing.

Perhaps if women were to have several lovers over their main sexual years they would in turn become better lovers themselves. A star tennis player is a star not only because of the inherent gift but also because that gift has improved with competition, regular practice and teaching.

Prostitutes are in regular practice. They have to please because they are being paid to do so, and if they aren't any good their upstairs competitor may filch customers and keep them. Prostitution is very competitive and pitches are jealously guarded. A prostitute isn't there to be upset over a poorly performing customer: it doesn't matter to her if he doesn't know what to do with his hands or if he's got bad cigarette breath, or even if his penis is on the small side and doesn't reach high enough inside her. Such inadequacies do matter, though, in a regular sexual partnership. Fat stomachs, hairy noses, long dirty nails, smelly breath and a poor idea of of ryhthm and timing are death to good sex.

I once knew a well-travelled attractive woman who was in a position to judge the sexual performance of a variety of men, including her husband and her one-night stands. She not only enjoyed each experience, just because she never knew what was coming next, but she enjoyed 'marking' their performance. The lowest mark she had ever given was a one out of ten! This man seemed fine on surface acquaintance, up to her normal social standards, but in bed, he just got it up and did nothing else with it. There was no movement, no change of positions, virtually no handwork anywhere and positively no talking. After just twenty minutes of lying there ready, at any stimulus, to churn into some of her own repertoire but not wishing to take over, she suddenly realized he was having an orgasm and that was that!

Having found a one out of ten, she realized two things. Firstly, that she certainly wasn't about to repeat the experience with him and secondly that her measurement yardstick now had both ends – one out of ten and ten out of ten.

The ten out of ten became, without any doubt, her husband. The immense love and sexual attraction they channelled into sex brought consistent peaks of fun and fulfilment. Sex at this level between them lasted any length of time from one to nine hours in any one session and then from nothing in a week to several times over a twenty-four-hour period. His penis was strong, sensitive, well controlled and cleverly used. He spent time, before and during, watching her body signals, talking and touching and bringing her to plateaus of pleasure until she was exhausted, and they were very much in love.

There was only one man ever to reach ten out of ten as well as her husband. He got his marking for a brilliant forty-minute body massage before two hours of sophisticated sexual skill that left her in a daze for three days! It appeared that he had enjoyed her, too, for he kept in contact by phone for some weeks and said that it was the best piece of sexual theatre he'd ever had. In between she apparently marked most men around the five to eight out of ten level.

Since, in general, women still do much of the responding, how are men to learn their own art? No night classes exist and even if they did, techniques alone, without natural flair and love, contain little spontaneous excitement. I sometimes wonder whether there could be value in getting two men to make love to a woman at the same time so they learn by comparing and suggesting and watching response levels. I suppose most women, like myself, would feel very uncomfortable in such a threesome even if it were at all possible to set up. Overall, I dare say, it wouldn't work, but how are men to be made better in bed? How can they improve to become eight, nine or ten?

Just taking twenty minutes for aiming at orgasm isn't making love. Twenty minutes of ramrod thrusting by a young man is one of the two major reasons for sexual cystitis, the other being poor hygiene mostly by the woman herself. This is explained later. For now, I want to concentrate on the ways in which men, through sexual activity, can cause cystitis in the female partner.

The rigidity of young men between nineteen and thirty-nine is not dissimilar to a broomhandle. The erect penis is as hard as wood. It widens as the years go by but it also softens up a bit. I'm told that in youth it almost burns with the sensation of wanting to get inside a female and that once there it feels as though it will burst open as sperm pressure builds up. The actual spurt of sperm is an enormous relief and the male can be weakly vulnerable and collapsed for a short time.

Very approximately, an erect male penis curves upwards, but if you were to stand ten naked erect men in a row and study this curve there would be differences. Some won't curve at all but point straight out at a right angle away from themselves. Others will have a left or right bearing and naturally the lengths will be different. Others will curve slightly inwards.

The vagina almost corresponds to the curving, but with a younger couple – he'll be at his most rigid and she'll be at her tightest – there's not a lot of room for easy movement. The vagina's capability of elasticity is potentially great, but before childbirth the muscles are very tight and not so yielding which means that they can bruise rather than absorb the impact. Think of a pair of shoes: they feel a bit close fitting when you try them on and wear them for the first time, but eventually they ease and when you finally throw them out they are probably loose!

If one sexual partner's penis is skewwhiff and doesn't roughly conform to your internal shape, it is possible that the thrusting will be skewwiff as well and not cleanly up and down the gap between the vaginal walls. It is to account for this sort of situation as well as the normal penile curve that position changing is healthy. Bruising is reduced on one sole area and the whole vagina absorbs the action, not just, say, the top left corner or the back wall. Changing the positions can mean simply shifting a bit more weight to one side by an inch or so. It doesn't just mean leaping around the bed and doing an Olga Korbut!

Young Lovers

'Honeymoon cystitis' or 'The Brides' Disease' as it was once called in the days when honeymoons were real, was purely caused by energetic penile thrusting into a narrow, ribbed vagina. You try banging your calf muscle with a broom handle for twenty minutes and see if it doesn't go pink, red or purple! You will also be going pink, red or purple inside, but it's impossible to see it. The smooth unmuscular cervix takes the brunt of the bruising and may ache for a day or so but if you get hold of a mirror and lie down you will certainly be able to see how the vaginal entrance and the vulva as a whole looks. Look at how the urethral opening is also discoloured and swollen.

The stinging feeling as you pass urine down the urethra soon after intercourse will be better next morning. The swelling inside is not only confined to the vagina but will be affecting all sorts of places you wouldn't think of. The urethra certainly swells and has been just as pummelled as the vagina, which is why it stings when acid urine tries to flow down the gap between the swollen urethral walls.

After intercourse, there's a lot of swollen skin outside and inside which starts to shade into a maroony and brown colour after a night's sleep. That night's rest is quite vital. The swollen skin is allowed to relax totally, the muscles don't even have to react to walking and so

110

they heal that much faster. The swelling recedes and any soreness dwindles away.

The uterus (womb) may ache a little because the thrusting of the head of the penis onto the cervix may have involved the cervical canal and uterus behind. If you are close to a period the whole thing is more sensitive because the lining of the uterus is already heavy with gathered blood. Intercourse on the first day of a period is naturally a bit messy, but it may be helpful in easing the period pain. It should be far gentler than normal with no deep positions and no heavy thrusting. Rhythmical relaxing and suctioning type movements can assist the early congestion as a lot of blood tries to escape down the cervical canal into the vagina. Bear down gently at times and at others go quiet for a moment to feel the vagina open wider.

Put lots of dark towels on the bed, make sure the room is nice and warm so that all top bed clothes can be thrown off and not get spoiled. Intercourse at this time is an individual choice, but generally it takes place within a relationship of great intimacy, one that is totally committed to a love of each other's body. There are men who adore intercourse at this time, and they would be best advised to use a sheath or certainly to pass urine and wash the foreskin (if uncircumcised) and penis in the shower afterwards. Blood is a culture medium for bacteria which is why many religions forbid intercourse for the whole seven days until the woman has douched and cleansed her vagina at the end.

If you are a young slim girl and your partner a young man who has a 'broomhandle' for a penis, some further thought on counteracting the effects of him may be helpful if you are sore afterwards or are, sadly, getting cystitis just from the bruising. Being slim is naturally always attractive, but being *thin* is different. You will be thin internally as well. Thin skin bruises more easily and so a vagina with thin skin layers may not protect the urethra adequately during intercourse. The bruised urethral nerve endings may start symptoms of urethritis and cystitis but without bacteria. Simply eating more, exercising less to encourage an extra six to ten pounds in weight may be an enormous help, if not the whole answer for many young women.

If you are young and unmarried, try first to select a place and a time where time, with a capital T, is available. I do realize this is often impossible but if I've pointed out the importance of time to you maybe you can organize it with some planning. You also need an empty building, so you relax totally and make a noise if you feel like it. Years ago fields and hedgerows were the best places but fields and hedgerows don't exist in huge towns and inner cities. Come to think of it, thanks to desert landscape farming, there aren't a lot of hedgerows left in the country even for the animals and birds, never mind lovers!

Always make sure you have to hand a box of tissues, a tube of lubricating jelly, a bath towel, an empty soda bottle for washing the perineum, another smaller towel to dry with, and check if he's likely to bring his own condom. *Don't* put the telly on. It's the greatest sex killer of all time! Put a nice supper together – the snacky sort not a great heavy meal, throw a cassette in the music centre, a candle in the holder and relax. I once had a session to remember forever, thanks to the trombones and kettledrums of the Women's Royal Army Corps band playing on a summer's afternoon on the bandstand below the hotel! Use all unusual circumstances – life's happiest memories can be made of such and they really don't happen that often.

If your boyfriend is more than casual and you have settled into a good steady affair, being as sure as you can be that he's not having it off with anyone else, have a go with the vaginal sponge instead of the condom by way of ringing the changes. That way you will both take a fair share of the responsibility.

If you are not completely relaxed you may not always be well lubricated. Perhaps you've had a tiring day, or you weren't well last night and didn't sleep properly. Such things can affect the amount of vaginal lubricant you secrete. It's nothing to worry about, but if your boyfriend's broomhandle is to slide in and out with as low a risk of damaging the vagina as possible, some KY jelly will come in handy.

KY jelly is obtainable without prescription from all pharmacies. Put a good dollop on your fingers – dollops not smears – maybe your boyfriend would like it on his fingers so that he can get some finger and hand practice. Tell him if he's hurting you anywhere but otherwise aim at gently massaging the vulva, clitoris and vagina with the lubricant. There's nothing like vaginal wetness to drive a man crazy with delight and if you've started out a bit on the dry side, the instant wetness will relax your mind away from all fear of bruising and soreness. The vagina will respond and start churning out more of its own liquid and, before you know it, five minutes have passed and you'll be reaching for the bath towel. Double it up and make sure it is well placed underneath, especially towards the backbone because liquids run along the seam of the perineum and gravity drops it off well past all the openings leaving an embarrassing stain or puddle somewhere.

Now's your chance, before penetration, to learn some sexual skill. When I was a drama student at Guildhall in London, we used to spend many hours each week in our curriculum doing things called improvizations – impros for short. These impros were unscripted dramatizations of any given situation, such as six people sitting in a railway carriage and the train hits the buffers. The dialogue and actions interact as each person gets an idea and others build on so that thirty to forty minutes of unscripted work flies by.

Sex is like this. One person tries something, the other reacts. The reaction brings more action and a whole interplay begins between the two people involved. Young lovers are usually both inexperienced and underskilled. The 'wanting' of each other, the urgency to penetrate, brings only a brief physical satisfaction of minutes. There's much extra satisfaction to be had from interplay and orchestration. Confidence builds up over the months as does the need for more sex because the hormone levels increase and encourage you to feel sexier. If you've got plenty of time, use outside influences like music, candles, a lacy half-slip, perfume, (if you're not allergic to it, and likely to sneeze), suspenders, a pretty necklace, change the place you generally have sex; lie down, sit down, stand up, bend over, tell stories (not fibs), recount a special sexual moment. Don't always aim for the orgasm at the end. Young men can, over several hours of sex, have between two and four full ejaculations, so whilst you discover each other by watching and listening, make sure, too, that you each look to the enjoyment of your own body every now and then.

The basic message is that the more relaxed and wet the vagina is, the less likely it is to sustain really painful bruising which may lead to cystitis.

Short, strong sexual sessions without stopping for a breather can cause awful bruising. The vagina must be allowed to stretch open for a minute or two after penetration. Lengthy sexual sessions, really lengthy, like over two hours, have to be accompanied by interludes of talking, resting, drinking and more KY jelly. Position changing is really important here and so delightful!

Go to the loo when you want, don't hold it because you're too embarrassed. Then fill the empty soda bottle with very cool water, and, after passing urine to ease the swollen urethra and expel any bacteria which may have found their way into the urethral opening, stay sitting on the lavatory whilst you pour the cool water down over the perineal openings. This water cools the swollen skin and reduces inflammation. Pat it gently, but very thoroughly, dry. Then having passed out the urine there will be less pressure on the vagina and uterus once you are penetrated again.

If you've got all this time planned out for a whole night you can afford to come back to bed and have a glass of something to replace the sweated and excreted body fluid. It's important for the kidneys not to become dehydrated at any time and it's important to make up liquid lost during any sort of exercise.

Energetic sex is one hell of an exercise! Both of you will be wonderfully sweaty and the bed quite damp. Take up a jug of iced water or orange squash for the two of you, no juices and nothing too sweet in case thrush might be encouraged. Alcohol can be drunk if you like, but do so sensibly.

Being stoned will not bring satisfaction. No star can perform well in any skill if rhythms are interrupted by drunken lurching. No, the use of alcohol in sex is best described, would you believe, by Jean Plaidy in one of her early historical novels. She puts Mary, Queen of Scots on a thick rug by a blazing Scottish log fire in a draughty castle bedroom and as Bothwell leans over her to start making love he takes a mouthful of full bodied wine and dribbles it into Mary's chattering mouth to warm her up!

I read that when I was quite a young teenager and to this day I remember it. It involves the lips and mouth, which are highly erotic areas, and, as the wine runs down the throat, the warmth spreads inside you, much as from the other end of the body, the penis spreads deeper in the vagina, and this way there's more heightened pleasure than just gulping from a glass. The biggest bonus is that you stop thinking of alcohol as a drink to be drunk. It can become yet another sexual pleasure to add to the repertoire. Two or three mouthfuls are enough.

A warning: mouths and throats are not always well. Don't kiss if you have a cold sore, don't use your tongues if either has a sore throat, cold, mouth thrush or any kind of sinusitus, tonsilitis or mouth infection. It really isn't fair to pass it on. Aids, we are warned, can be passed through the wet medium of any bodily mucous. Make absolutely certain of the trustworthiness of your partner. I'm much afraid that we may all have to get used to regular blood tests and to showing the results, on headed medical reports, to a new sexual partner. It sounds like a Hollywood fantasy, doesn't it, but it's very real.

The positions of sex are very varied, as the amazing Kama Sutra and various Greek frescoes show. I think the climate is the major influence myself: a cold room spells restricted activity; a really warm room spells abandon!

I find it interesting that men don't go on these days about their wives being frigid. Perhaps in the light of good public communications on sexual matters they feel that this, supposed frigidity could rebound on themselves as being poor lovers. On the other hand, it's quite possible that the advent of central heating in most homes means warmer bedroom and warmer women. Women sometimes feel the cold more than men, and it only takes five minutes of the more static female role in the missionary position to reduce her to a shivering unresponsiveness.

She'll be constantly pulling up the bedclothes, wanting to wear a nightie and generally wrecking the whole business by asking if he's come yet. There's no way in a cold room that you can practice any sexual finesse. Breasts may well tighten and nipples go hard which men find very exciting, but if she's tight and dry in the vagina, as well she may be, penetration will be trickier. It only needs three or four unsuccessful pushes at the vaginal entrance

116

by a 'broomhandle' to make the vaginal muscles resentful and tight. Increased pressure to attain penile entry will tear the entrance, especially at the side nearest the back passage. That's where the perineal seam is at its tightest and most resistant. Once there's a tiny tear, intercourse for that session will be unpleasurable for the female. She will be aware and thinking of every thrust and whether the tear will hurt or get worse.

Bacteria, if present, will gain ready entrance through the tear and she may now face a twofold problem – the pain and soreness of the injury itself, plus infection. If this has happened before she'll also add fear to her trouble. The trouble could be likely to range from two or three days of ordinary soreness – stinging on the tear as urine touches it – or it could go all the way to a big attack of bladder cystitis, not just urethral cystitis. Any of this she will learn to dread.

Several months of such misery will removed thoughts of sex as a pleasure from her. Her fear and dread will rub off and affect her partner. It doesn't take my writing here to let you imagine the far-reaching, long-term results of such trouble: sexual separation, distress, rows, doctors, investigations, separate bedrooms, sexual infidelity and total break up of the relationship.

All from a cold bedroom I hear you say? Certainly, and the group most at risk are the young lovers where social conditions are less stable than in a homely place where heating can be controlled and maintained by the lovers themselves to their own requirements.

I had a young woman for counselling who was living with her boyfriend in his flat. He liked a cold bedroom and, being an economic bloke as well, turned his heating off well in advance of bedtime. This meant that the bathroom was cold too. She survived the bedroom but admitted not doing the bottle washing afterwards because she was too cold to go into the bathroom. Often she wouldn't bother to pass urine either and so was lining up her cystitis quite easily with sex, having read another of my books. Her cystitis only ever happened after sex, and sometimes the lab tests on her urine sample showed positive infection, but sometimes not.

She knew the reason why she neglected her hygiene after sex and her boyfriend knew perfectly well that she was chilly but neither had fully acknowledged the tremendous importance of room temperatures until my counselling spelled it out. Keep the heating on, so that bedroom and bathroom are nice and warm. Then apply lubricating jelly liberally before and during intercourse as necessary, pass urine and bottle wash as specified.

Once you have surrounding warmth, it becomes so much easier to change from one sexual position to another. For instance, the whole of the bed, its end and wall and its other three edges can all become theatrical props. You don't *have* to lie in the sleeping situation of head at the top, feet at the bottom of the bed. You don't *have* to lie down at all! You can sit, kneel, bend over both on the bed and its edges. Flicking through just one copy of *Playboy* or *Penthouse* will spark of enough ideas for your own improvisation to last forever. Hard porn is very distasteful and quite unnecessary, mostly because you'll get far better kicks from your own inventions and also because being in a love/sex relationship rather than a straight sex one will discard the degradation associated with porn. Those films and magazines are not promoting love, they're promoting fortunes. Why make that sort of rich man richer?

If you are starting out on your sex life and reading this, can I recommend you to buy Dr David Delvin's *Book of Love*. He and his illustrators, Patricial Quayle and Ray Feibush, have put together good sensitively drawn ink sketches of sexual positions.

For young 'broomhandles' and slim vaginas I think the

following positions can be tried, with care and yelled warnings if anything hurts! Dull, pleasurable ache is one thing, strong internal pain quite another.

Handwork, as I prefer to call it rather than masturbation, will relax and enlarge the vagina, but the young 'broomhandle' needs little, if any, handwork to become excited. The young male usually needs holding back so that he's not a disappointment – which means that whilst he would be ecstatic with any handling or oral work on his penis he's likely to blow a fuse and turn the lights out too early!

Not to worry if that happens! It can be very exciting to have a man absolutely unable to control himself because you are so provocative, and if he is that excited, he'll probably be growing hard again in twenty or thirty minutes for a steadier and more prolonged intercourse. In the meantime have a good cuddle. Women love that and adore being held closely. It's something many men don't understand, but I maintain that they don't need to understand it, just knowing it, accepting it and doing it should be enough.

Do to each other anything that you both enjoy, except touching or penetrating the anus. It is perfectly possible to spend hours caressing, stroking, massaging any part of each other's body, and particularly inside the vagina.

Which sort of hand would stroke best? I know what I'd prefer and which sort I'd trust not to infect me or set up a skin reaction. Only a clean, scrubbed and well-rinsed hand should go near sensitive genitalia. If your partner usually likes some handwork, don't put hand cream on before you work on him, it may contain some chemical that could cause allergic reaction. Rinsed hands and a lot of KY will do nicely. This is a sterile, non-greasy variety.

If non-bacterial cystitis is playing a part in association with sex, have a think about where hands are for most or part of the day. Have you really got rid of the coal dust

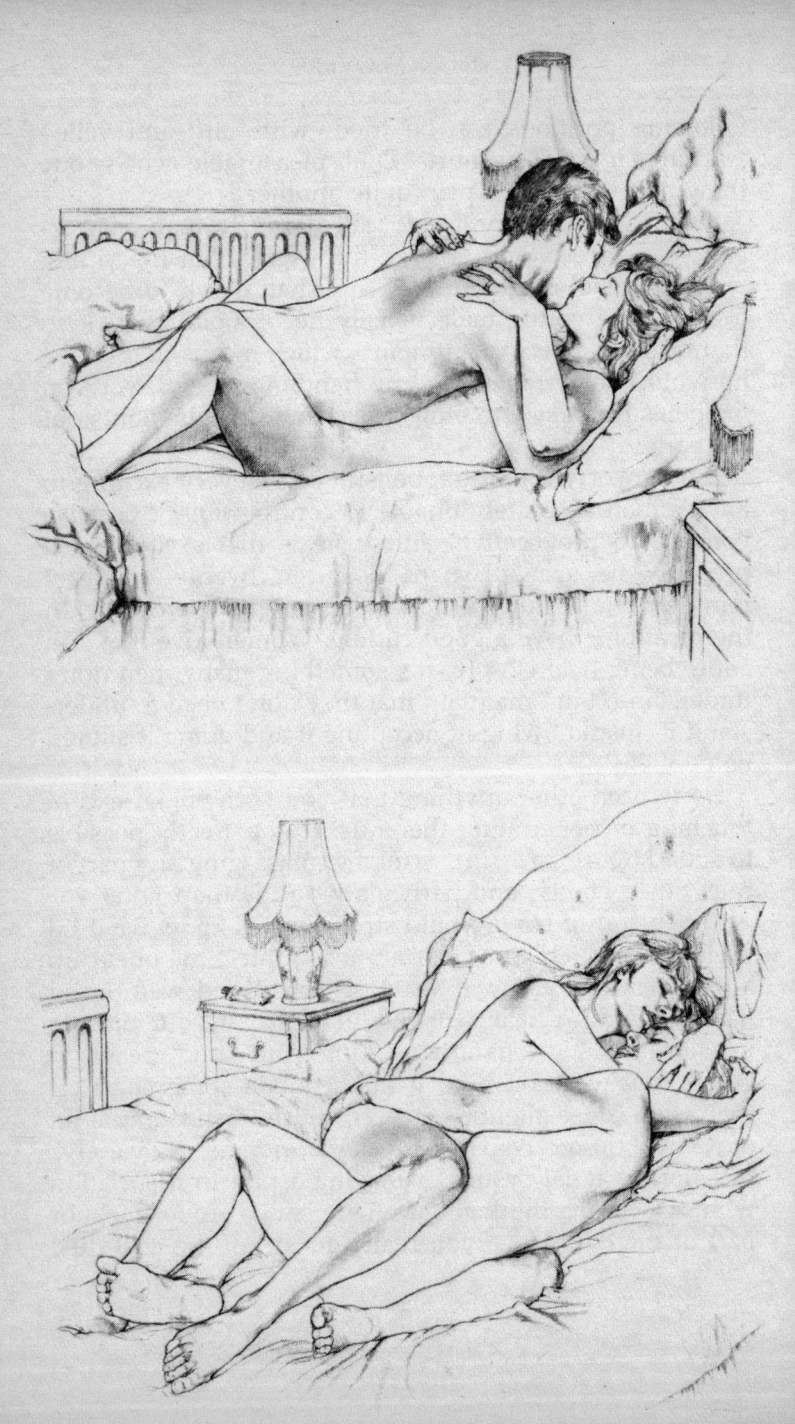

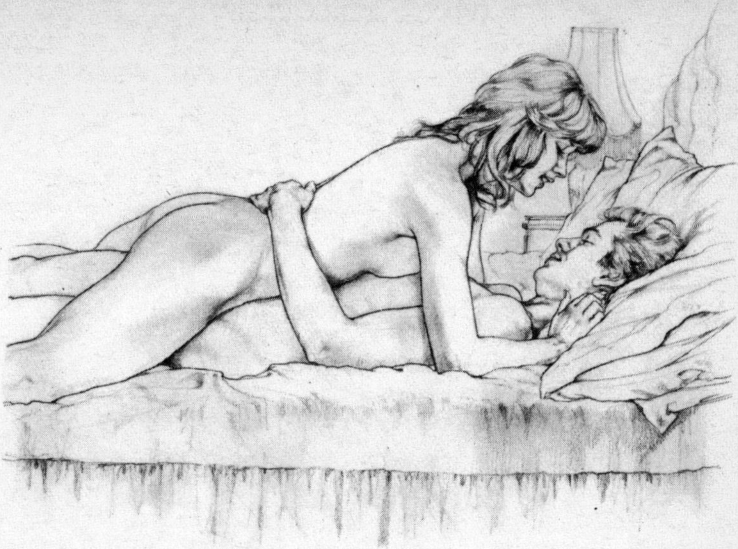

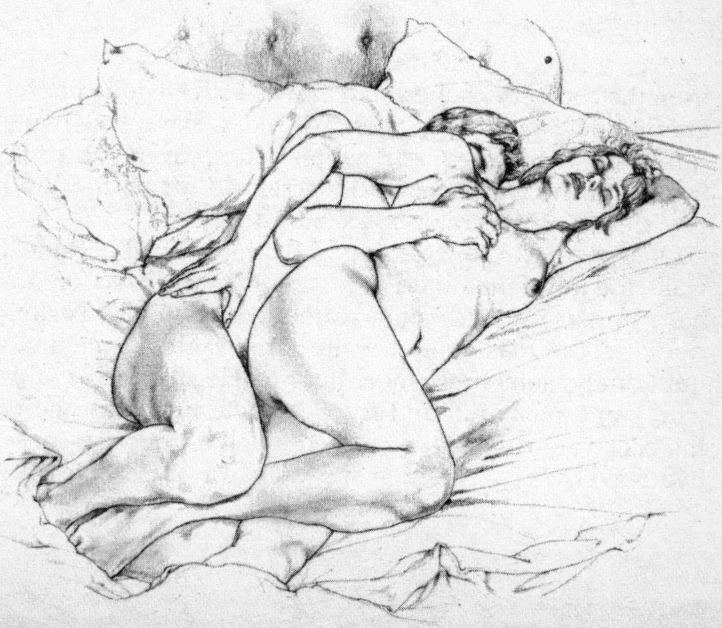

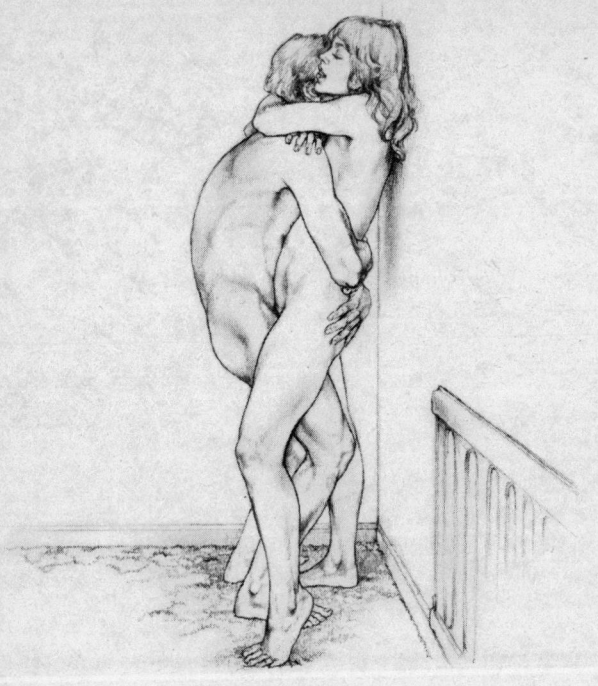

from the coalmine, have you really de-activated the photographic developer from the dark room, have you really rinsed off the 'Rose Clear' when you sprayed the roses before lunch? Have you really scrubbed off all the sand particles from the children's sand pit?

One good way of opening and preparing the vaginal walls for full penetration is for the man to insert one or more fingers into the vagina, carefully and slowly. Feeling round he can massage the walls of the vagina, sometimes flutteringly, sometimes more heavily. He should vary this with some push/pull and try also some firm massage of the back vaginal wall which then involves the very sensitive bowel walls. The opposite vaginal wall contains the

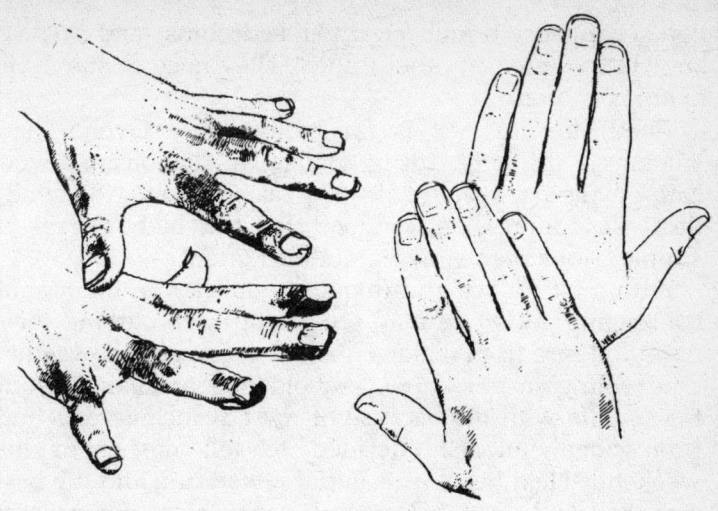

Hands should be clean, scrubbed and well-rinsed, with fingernails filed smooth. Dirty hands with broken fingernails can irritate and injure the vagina

body or root of the clitoris and if the male gets his fingers on that just right and uses just the right amount of firmness and rhythm, the female may produce a really good orgasm. Practice makes perfect and a towel will be needed. The whole object is to reduce the possibility of vaginal bruising and non-bacterial sexual cystitis.

If she really lets go and has a big orgasm there's a chance, unless she's well practiced at controlling it, that the urethra may spasm as well and allow urine to escape. There's no perversion in this, it's just physiologically unavoidable. Sometimes she may not want this and if she's really determined will seize the hand and force it to a halt.

Sex, with health and cleanliness is the best possible sort of sex. Women have far more intercourse now than they did forty or fifty years ago. That has to do with contraception, changed attitudes, warmer bedrooms, and greater knowledge amongst other things. They need to stay well to enjoy it often.

Good, healthy sex is far better for everyone than smoking, drinking, drug-taking, workaholism, over-eating, jogging, keep fit. Healthy sex is good for the mind, decreases depression; is good for the body, keeps it supple; stops men straying quite so often!

With a bit of luck and frequent publicity on the fear of contracting Aids, we may see young men curbing their natural desire from making a rut at every passing vagina. One young man I know, emboldened at talking about his sex life with me because of my advancing years and professional interest, decided to tell me about his weekend. He'd been an usher at a wedding and the best man had laid on (what a pun!) some 'birds' for each of the ushers since they were all away from home territory for the weekend. So my young friend was more than happy to fall in with the plans and had obviously enjoyed it. The 'bird' allotted to him was obviously the easygoing type. So without nagging or being clever, I asked straight off if she'd told him who had been lying on top of her the previous night or the last Saturday night. It stopped him dead and I said that I supposed he'd never bothered to think about that. But since she was obviously without any reticence, she'd done it so often that she had no moral qualms or knowledge of disease. Was such easy, casual sex likely to be a hundred per cent healthy? And how did he, my friend, know forty-eight hours later that he hadn't caught anything? He hadn't used a condom. Enough said. He came a week later saying, as any sensible young man should, that he'd given some thought to what I had said and decided I was right. He'd be more choosy and careful.

A good lesson for everybody!

Sex In Pregnancy

I'm going to start this section with pregnancy and child-birth, mostly to get it out of the way! There are many books dealing in general with sex and foetal development, but my idea is to give you a few tips to help you avoid cystitis at such times. The first thing to remember is that cystitis by itself is no barrier to conceiving a child. If your cystitis is part of other symptoms sugesting hormone deficiencies, pelvic disorder, Fallopian or ovarian obstructions then you wouldn't be likely to conceive anyway.

Ordinary cystitis, with or without bacteria, will not stop conception. Many a woman has confided her worry about (a) conceiving, and (b) coping with the continuing cystitis as well as the pregnancy, delivery and aftercare of herself and her baby.

Every pregnancy is an individual affair. Until it starts, it will be impossible for anyone to predict how your body is going to behave. So no-one can advise or recommend in advance. Pregnancy symptoms can range from nothing at all to increased nasal congestion, increased vaginal discharges, haemorrhoids, morning sickness, nausea, itchy thigh skin, swollen breasts, heartburn, glossier hair, no cystitis, less cystitis, more cystitis, first-time cystitis, urinary frequency, swollen ankles, increased sexual

125

desire, decreased sexual desire, high blood pressure, and a multitude of horriblenesses.

A lot of hereditary tendencies are implanted within the conceived embryo: hair colour for instance, skin sensitivity for instance, and physiological sensitivities. Lung troubles are often hereditary: couldn't some forms of cystitis be hereditary? It could be, but I find that it mostly isn't. Again remember that cystitis is only a symptom of another basic condition. I always probe further if a patient in counselling volunteers that her mother, grandmother or sisters have also known cystitis. There's a case in my book, *Victims of Thrush and Cystitis*, which touches on this, and, certainly for a lot of women I've met over the years, there has been a past generation link. What I have never done is take a full case history from such related women. One day maybe! If I was, at this stage in my knowledge, to hazard a guess, I'd still go along with things like skin sensitivity, background allergies, womanly household traditions and hormone patterns.

This can be complicated by the hereditary tendency skipping a generation or missing the opposite sex. I think my own allergic sensitivities come from two sides, with only very mild manifestations in my own mother and father. But I'm sure that neither of my grandmothers had honeymoon conditions like mine. I'm sure they had no swimming, no wine with each meal, no vaginal foam contraceptive, no nylon swimsuit, no hot dehydrating sunbathing, no heavy sex, no spicy hot food. Therefore probably no cystitis, but they were old ladies during my own years of cystitis and I'd never have thought of asking them about it because I was so ignorant. To my personal knowledge, no member of my family anywhere has any experience of cystitis bar the one short attack my mother had when she was in her sixties.

My daughter, the next generation, had one attack in very early childhood due to hexachlorophane contamination of her entire vulval area when I washed her hair in the bath regularly with a medicated shampoo. Since then, all has been well and if *she* has a ruined honeymoon too, I shall scream!

My cystitis completely stopped in my first pregnancy (I didn't get it in my second one five years later, either, but by then I'd stopped the attacks myself outside of the pregnancy with self-help). Neither I nor my doctors had a reason to offer for its disappearance at that time, and I just thanked God for nine months' relief. After that first pregnancy, from August 1968 to May 1969, I returned to the same hellish state until seeing Mr Shuttleworth in March 1970 when slowly, so slowly, I began to learn that I myself could take charge and prevent cystitis attacks. I thanked God for Mr Shuttleworth, too, and his first mention of passing urine after intercourse.

I know plenty of women who get their first ever attacks in pregnancy and I've written in detail in *Understanding Cystitis* of some of the medical reasons for this. There are still things like increased normal vaginal discharges which irritate the urethral opening but which can be easily cleaned out by the patient, and once a swab has been lab tested for offending bacteria and found to be unresponsible for the secondary cystitis symptoms, you can increase your vigilance with the bottle washing. Be especially careful about scrubbing fingers and nails before hooking out the discharge from the vagina. Again a reminder not to put any kind of soap on the vulva, but only plain water poured out of the bottle as you sit well back on the lavatory. (No bidets, remember!) This will remove the itchy, but non-bacterial discharge and stop it being massaged up the urethra when you sit or walk. Go without underwear to keep the perineum dry and healthy. Do fight the urge to wear dungarees. It is far healthier to wear a long skirt or caftan because you will discourage the increased possibility of candida growth.

If you get bacterial cystitis which has been properly diagnosed from a urine test, take the antibiotics prescribed, ask for vaginal pessaries to counteract any predisposition to vaginal thrush and eat plenty of live yoghurt before meals to encourage lactobacillus to fight full body thrush.

If the urine test shows any bowel bacteria to be responsible (ask your GP about the origin of the bacteria if you're not sure) for the pregnancy cystitis, just check on the state of your anus. Have you got any skin tabs or external piles that can be harbouring germs? You should then be even more stringent about the bottle washing if bacteria are found.

Re-check all your actions after a bowl movement. If the normal times at which you empty your bowels have changed, think about any effect from that, or maybe the stool is more frequent and almost diarrhoea. Are you washing after each movement? You must! Don't strain away when you are pregnant if the stool has become more solid. Take a safe laxative, eat stewed apples every other day (don't over acidize the urine!) and ask the pharmacist for a good anti-haemorrhoid suppository, or mention the problem to the GP if it really is bothersome.

Bowels and bladder will be working for the two of you, so don't worry about passing more urine or more faecal material. Don't hold the urine back and try not to let the bowels become congested or the stools will be wider and more difficult to expel.

I know that since the thalidomide tragedy, pregnant women have been very scared of any drug, even if it's non-prescribable, but equally if you have an illness or infection in pregnancy and you let it spread untreated, this can be just as detrimental to the baby. Take what medication you must. Your GP will be just as aware as you are but may be able to allay your fears on any pharmacological product and help you get better so that you can enjoy your pregnancy.

During pregnancy you will want to continue intercourse. Go ahead. It must be made very plain to your husband that a shower each evening is great protection against vaginal infections or inflammations and that his nails and hands must be scrupulous, too. All for the baby's benefit. He should be doing it for your benefit anyway.

Penetration from behind is more comfortable, especially after the fourth or fifth month. Curl up and let him gently reach to the depth inside which you instinctively feel is not going to hurt either you or the baby. He should then move the rest of his body to account for that depth as he starts rhythmic pushing, and not overreach to where you would feel uncomfortable.

If you aren't too large yet, lie on your back, put one pillow in a position underneath you which will elongate your pelvis and let the baby move with gravity up a little to your waist. Your husband may then insert all his penis if he kneels between your legs and supports himself with sturdy arms. Try asking him to go his whole penile length slowly in and then out until the tip of the penis is virtually out but just stops the vaginal entrance from closing up before moving in again. A few slow pushes and withdrawals of this kind with the baby between you will bring sheer joy. It's not enough movement to bruise and all sex in pregnancy should be non-bruising.

If he's extra aroused by your forthcoming motherhood he may well be wanting to ejaculate externally almost anywhere on you. Let him. Help him ejaculate, it may be a new experience and one which you can add to the skill repertoire. You might invent a little competition for yourself with the digital watch to see how fast you can make him come and the fastest or slowest he took in the nine months. Use the sperm fluid instead of jelly for a massage. An hour or so of this kind of sex will soon show

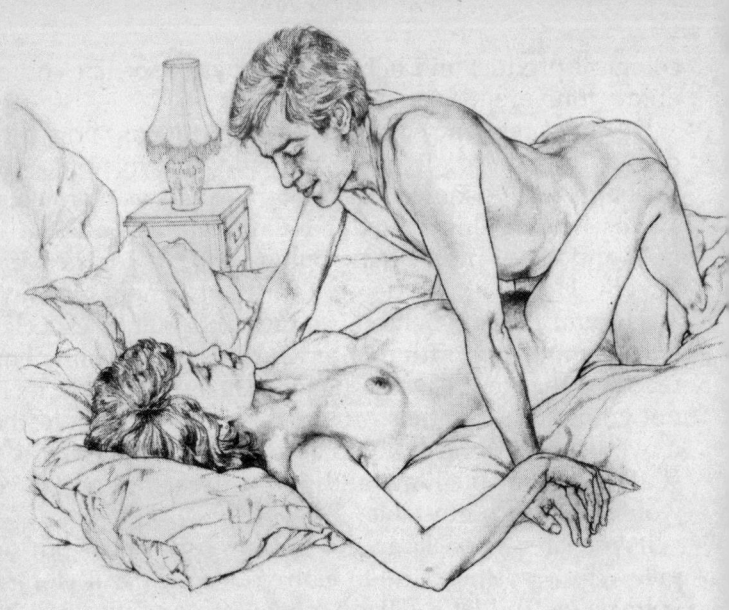

a decrease in TV football viewing figures! Much handwork is recommended in pregnancy, not just because of impeded penetration but because there are new things to feel and marvel at. If he feels you, you feel him and butter up his ego with talk of fruitful loins and seeds and things. He'll love it! Your bodies exist for the enjoyment of both of you, and you should both revel in this nine months worth of extended arousal.

Penile entry of the vagina from the rear in pregnancy is one of nature's protections. The penis moves in such penetration in a frontal direction whilst the baby stays in the body of the pelvic cavity – except it does spread everywhere from the seventh to the ninth month! Try kneeling, with your head on the bed perhaps holding one or two pillows under the neck and breasts. Very gently get him also to kneel and feel the penis slowly in. The baby has again dropped a bit towards your waist with

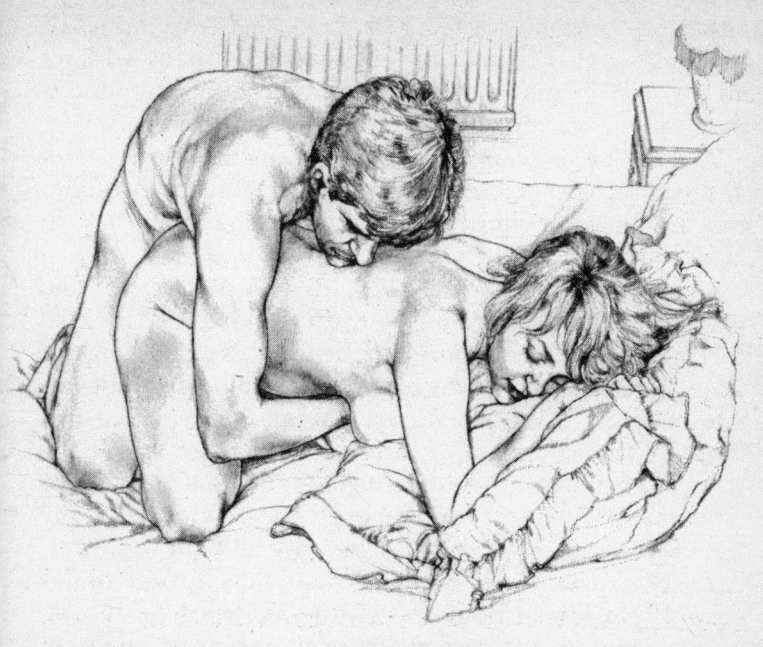

gravity, your buttocks will take away a bit of the penile length and the vagina will lengthen. Any pushing must be dictated by your comfort so don't tense. Actively relax and open up, having been reassured that he's not going to go berserk and rape you!

The more your husband is allowed inside you, the more he'll get to know your comfort levels and the more you can relax and enjoy it. Familiarity breeds pleasure here, not contempt. Earlier bedtimes will help so that time is with you not against you.

Second and subsequent pregnancies may renew the old excitements but if you were unlucky with scarring and had to have a wretched episiotomy, there may be a bit more sensitivity and possibility of scar tear. Lubricating jelly is the key in such difficulties. Avoid bearing down either in orgasm, plateau orgasms, passing urine or passing faecal material. If your husband is handworking you, you'll have to explain the scar and how easily it can nick so that he can work around the tender spot.

A second episiotomy can make for much misery in bed and be an easy source of discomfort, trauma or infection. Discuss the scar with a good gynaecologist and try to avoid having it re-opened.

Having a baby is part of sex – the end product and the beginning of a new era for your own body. Poor medical care in the delivery room, particularly over sewing up tears, internally and externally, can account for a never-ending cycle of sexual misery. If, and it's a huge if – because there's sadly so little medical attention to the new mother's comfort immediately after delivery in big hospitals – if you can just ignore your new cuddly baby for a few minutes and consult with the midwife or doctor, you should do so. It is better right now to put things correctly inside and out and ensure, as best you all can, a return to a healthy trouble-free vagina and perineum. If after six weeks, when you have an an internal checkup jagged scars, flaps of skin, or loose stitching are found it will mean more time spent at hospital or simply putting up with the effects.

Ask the gynaecologist for some sort of anaesthetic so that he can do a careful unhurried repair now. A whiff of gas and air may help for smaller exernal work, but create a fuss if you can see that they are aiming to stitch a lot and get away without using an anaesthetic. Don't ever let anyone try to hold or strap you down, it's barbaric and smacks of Dr Mengele. If you wriggle they can't stitch properly and so it's worth their while as well as yours to have good pain reduction.

If you have a sensitive skin then request the mildest possible antiseptic solution for swabbing. Plain water will do well enough until the first salt bath and should help to avoid a rash or further soreness.

During one of my own children's birth I was catheterized. We had all decided previously that because of my bladder history it should be avoided unless absolutely necessary. Well, a very lengthy and tiring birth made it necessary and, sure enough, thirty-six hours later came the first twinges of cystitis. The first in three years. I asked for a urine test and started some antibiotics. The test result came back with E. Coli and I can remember being amazed at an infection starting in hospital amidst what I thought would be stringent hygiene.

My gynaecologist also dealt with some anal skin tabs whilst I took a whiff of the gas machine and he performed an episiotomy some minutes later. In vaginal birthing the perineal skin can be strained to tearing point and when I began to split he neatly knifed rather than let me tear untidily. The third thing to happen was the catheterization up the urethra to let out gathering urine which was becoming an impediment. The catheterizing alone could have introduced infection but possibly the anal and perineal knifing allowed easy passage along the cut for anal bacteria which could have been massaged up the urethra on the surface of the catheter tube.

Bacterial cystitis after delivery is not uncommon. Take your washing bottle to the hospital so that you can wash the perineum down just as though you were at home. After passing a stool, be very thorough so that anal bacteria can't get a hold in the damaged and bruised perineal skin. Make sure you line the hospital loo seat in the front with paper so that infection risk is reduced.

Wear a loose sanitary towel, and if you are in bed don't bother to do it up over the pubic hair. Make sure that it is well placed at the back so that gravitational drainage is caught. If you lie with just the sheet over you and your legs bent, the perineum will cool and heal faster and the weight will be taken off the bruised vulva as well.

I'm not in favour of too many hot salt baths. The value of the salt is not denied, it's the doubtful value of the hot water when you are already swollen that I question. Bottle washing is still preferable so when you wash the perineum down after passing a stool pop some salt in the bottle for a final rinse off.

Talking of the salt reminds me of the day in the Holloway Road Sainsbury's where the man in front of me at the checkout queue had twenty-six one-kilo packets of table salt. There was some speculation round about and a few women close by, including me, were quite giggly. Finally, me being me, just had to ask if he kept a pig farm and was intending to salt down a lot of bacon. 'No', he said seriously, 'my wife's just had a baby and the hospital says she's got to have a lot of salt baths.' Well, the place erupted!

'Did you say *a* baby? Not sextuplets?'

'That'll do her for four deliveries!'

'She'll be in salt baths till Christmas!'

It was a very funny moment.

If you have a *good* rest after a *good* delivery, and the most telling points of a return to normality are happening – no discomfort on passing urine; no discomfort on passing a stool; no further bleeding; sitting on chairs with ease - it may be hard to wait for six weeks before resuming intercourse. Try to hang on until six weeks because the cervix and uterus can't be aided by external cooling so they may still be not quite back to size.

Gentle exercises (you'll find some in *Understanding Cystitis*) will help flatten the abdominal muscles and tighten up the pelvic floor. They are important for the bladder and uterus because good, careful work on them now may prevent prolapse in later years. Prolapse operations, where they hitch up the bladder and/or the uterus, are never a hundred per cent successful and indeed the situation has to be quite bad in the first place before a surgeon will agree to operate.

Drink a fair amount to keep the bladder and urethra 'clean' and make every effort to excrete what you drink. Steer off sweetened drinks and juices except as real treats and watch out for all funny, yellow coloured drinks because the tartrazine doesn't agree with everyone. To much 'visitors" fruit like grapes, plums, strawberries etc., may acidize the urine and it will sting as it flows down a bruised urethra. Too much fruit will also give your baby diarrhoea if it's being breast-fed.

Lucky you, if intercourse is all right when it is resumed after six weeks. The sheath and withdrawal may be the contraceptives best used for a while; plenty of jelly, especially if you had an internal tear. Have a word with the gynaecologist at the checkup about contraceptives if you are breast-feeding. Some women go on the Pill once breast-feeding is secure but you are entitled to have your own ideas.

If penetration results in no adverse discomfort, pain or urinary involvement then it is safe to assume childbirth suits you. The amount of time taken by individual women to recover their full sexual health is variable. Judge your improvement on a regular basis and try to gauge if the discomfort is lessening. If it is slowly decreasing, nature is simply taking time – no doctor can possibly improve on the natural healing process so be patient. Any discharge or bleeding should be reported and another internal given.

Once you are fully recovered and sexual intercourse is back to its previous patterns there will be opportunities for new positions – the sort of third phase. Tiredness from twenty-four-hour babycare may take the edge off the length of time you make love but what you lose there you can make up with new variations. Use the breast-feeding times, if you are still doing that. Lie on your side to feed the baby, letting your husband join up from behind in bed at the night-time feed. Buy a comfy armchair of just the right height and design, which you can keep anywhere in the house – bedroom, sitting room, or elsewhere - then breast or bottle-feed in it and get your husband to kneel between your legs both for handwork or full penile movement. Use lubricating jelly if you're tired and dry to start with, and this will avoid aggravating any internal bruising left over from the birth. Don't go off sex just because you may not feel as wet as you did before the baby. It'll come back once you are sexually psyched up.

With a vagina that has full expansion ability after the child has arrived, there is no end to sexual positions. For instance, your husband may now be able to get three fingers inside and move them instead of two at a pinch; you will be able to bring both legs over his shoulders, an extremely deep entry and one which will become even more tolerable over the years as his rigidity declines. You may not yet feel like letting him move or thrust in this position, but wait till he's older!

Sitting astride him will still be more uncomfortable near a period but halfway through the cycle should find you able and willing to move on him. Once you're secure on top there are many simple enjoyments best left to other books or your own devising, but one day try turning yourself until you face his feet. This, too, is an extremely deep penetration and best done with care. It may feel difficult to make any movement so just handle him instead.

At times, because of his own tiredness from a heavy day, he will be less hard. It's this sort of occasion that lets you take a more active part. Use his body, he'll love that, and then freely explore any deeply penetrative positions that produce discomfort at other times. Don't worry, or, worse still, get him uptight about being softer. Be genuinely delighted – you ought to be anyway – that he's softer sometimes and you can explore deeper penetration.

Memories of good or unusual intercourse unimpeded by sexual cystitis are part of the stuff of life. Remember them and store them for your old age when one of you is gone. You may look back as a cystitis sufferer and find that cystitis due to bruising, trauma and nicking, slowly decreases over the years. This would be especially true for the generations who didn't have any books to help put them right in their youth, and for those generations that have been traditionally less sexually active.

Nuns don't get *sexual* cystitis, nor do any other celibate women. The more sexual activity you have the more likelihood there is of cystitis, urethritis, vaginitis, and many other conditions.

Sex in Later Life

The softer the penis becomes with advancing years the less chance there is of bruising and trauma in the female partner. 'Broomhandle' becomes a thing of the past. The slim ramrod expands in width, although it doesn't necessarily lose length. Correspondingly, the vagina will be losing its tight muscular tone. On no account does all this mean that pleasure is lost. For many people the pleasure heightens because sex is without discomfort. People in their fifties/sixties have skill, co-ordination, less fear of pregnancy, mobility, time on their side and more holidays.

The whole range of sexual positions becomes possible, though perhaps stale marriages, weary from child-rearing and career commitments, are not so conducive to a good bedroom romp. Revitalize your life with some mineral supplements, some weight reduction and maybe a treat week at a health farm. Go shopping for a new set of underwear and new sheets or take a weekend away. Whatever might turn you both on.

The most common sexual cause of cystitis, ranking equal with the bruising, is infection and this is now the more likely root cause in middle age and after if cystitis is only happening after intercourse. Your main proof is gleaned from urine test results. Ask for a vaginal swab at the same time to see if bacteria are present there also.

As vaginal health starts its gradual decline near, during and after menopause, the lining will be more prone to invasive bacteria and to dryness. Bacteria is still mostly coming from the bowel and by increasing perineal hygiene, you can sort that one. Dryness is treatable too. Simple sexual dryness will respond to lubricating jelly, but if the dryness is bordering on continual discomfort or burning, hormone treatment may be indicated.

Other symptoms of hormone imbalance include depression, lethargy, hot flushes, limb aches, cystitis and great vaginal discomfort. I've seen so many women aged between forty and eighty with these sorts of symptoms who have been under-treated with only smears of vaginal hormone cream. It seems to be hard for many gynaecologists to understand that hormones don't all congregate at the vaginal opening! Hormones are blood-borne and lack of them, like lack of minerals or vitamins, will make the patient feel awful. Read Wendy Cooper's wonderful *No Change*, published by Arrow Books.

Hormone treatment by mouth or by implant is necessary for lots of women now that we live longer. Find a meno-pause clinic (Wendy Cooper's book names a lot) or a gynaecologist whose life's work centres upon this area of women's health. Other gynaecologists are still backward in their appreciation of just how vital hormone treatment is for women. Improvement in attitude is happening but it's slow. Improvement of the imbalance can be very slow but it can also, with the implant system, be dramatic. Many patients feel a daily rise in the quality of life and diminution of symptoms and often, six weeks after the implant, they are new women. If an implant is rejected and oral tablet treatment used instead, patience and more patience and yet more patience may be required. Depending on the strength of the tablets, it could be six months before you feel halfway better.

Libido should improve with the decrease of vaginal

139

burning and discomfort. Gentle intercourse with plenty of jelly can be started again and slowly put back on the twice weekly evening diary. The more the ageing vagina is used the healthier it will be. I once sat next to a French gynaecologist at a dinner and we touched on hormone imbalance in our conversation. Whilst he used hormone treatment when absolutely necessary he maintained that regular intercourse was effective in counteracting ageing. He professed to making love to his attractive and elegant grey-haired wife as often as possible, and said that she had had a good menopause. Now in her sixties she certainly had a good glow on her and took great care with make-up and clothes. Her health was excellent for her age and she was obviously without sexual health problems or she couldn't have made love regularly. Are these two people just lucky, or have they worked hard to maintain their dual libido and dual sexual ability?

The ideal of marriage is to spend young, middle and old years together so that age creeps on slowly and with dignity. If the overall relationship stays happy, sexual happiness should go hand in hand, with intercourse remaining as one part of that overall happiness. Life isn't like that, though, for the majority, and such ideals are very hard to achieve. If doctors have to step in with replacement therapy to stop aches, pains and more severe symptoms like cystitis we should all be grateful that at least such therapy does exist.

Other Sorts of Sex

This book is not written to moralize. Nevertheless, public morality is often born out of centuries of revolving tradition. Much tradition is born out of practicality for the survival of the species. So we should ponder upon it. The love of one member of a sex for another member of the same sex will not promote survival of the human race. Homo and lesbian sexuality may therefore be described as without root or reason. Any anal intercourse between two people will not increase the population. Any use of the anus is a dangerous practice, carrying high risk of injury and disease.

Many partners now practise oral sex. Providing it is undertaken willingly and account is taken of the health of the teeth, mouth, throat and genitalia, it can be pleasurable.

If urethritis and/or cystitis occur in either partner within forty-eight hours of oral sex then it's important to go somewhere for penile, vaginal, and throat swabs. Urine samples from both partners are also necessary and, to oversee all this, it is preferable to use a VD or genito-urinary clinic where male and female sections are in the one department. If luck is on your side, the same doctor may even see you both.

The ready vision of oral sex is one of the male organ

in the female mouth, thanks to male sex industrialists, publishers and blue movie directors. In the private bedroom where degradation and dominance feature less, there is also emphasis on vulval stimulation and honest 'serving' by the male partner. I frequently turn to the sexuality of raw nature to see how males and females deal with copulatory traditions. I don't remember ever seeing or reading of the female of a given species licking the male organ of her mate. She certainly licks her offspring a great deal and will lick to clean its genitals if necessary. Mostly in animal sex the male will sniff and nuzzle the female organs when allowed the chance, not vice versa.

Actually, 'perversion' is missing in most private bedrooms. There is instead an intimate two-way traffic of tongues and mouths which decidedly gives a lot of pleasure to both people. Oral sex can be achieved both in a simultaneous act and separately. It helps greatly if you can both bath together first and actually witness the washing which promotes the confidence afterwards in trouble-free oral lovemaking. Don't put bubble baths in your bath water as they can cause urethritis.

Drying one another after a bath leads easily to licking. Stray drops of bath water are tempting to the eye and tongue and there's no part of the newly washed and scented body that seems uninviting. If vulval licking and kissing starts do make sure your partner knows the landscape of your vulva and that he realises tongues can be strong. If he employs a strong tongue or tight lips by mistake on the urethral opening, some sort of damage may result. A tiny nick or a graze from untended chin stubble could really cause trouble from urethritis and ascending cystitis if you're prone.

Rape

Rape as a cause of cystitis may now make sense to the reader but in the early 'seventies when I was beginning my U & I Club for cystitis sufferers, neither I nor the general multitude would have thought of an association between the two. The rape crisis centre was beginning its work for rape victims, and one day the director telephoned me for leaflets on how to deal with cystitis which I was then distributing. I sent them, of course, to anyone on request but I asked why the rape group would need leaflets on cystitis. I was told that awful urethral and bladder damage could result from violent penetration. And naturally, as a woman, it only needed that sentence for me to imagine what might happen.

The age of the victim is immaterial. That she may be skilled and well practised at breathing deeply and expanding her vagina counts for nothing in the state of panting fear induced by threatened and real physical violence.

At every turn the victim's fear produces immense tension in the pelvis and that tension removes the elasticity necessary for internal organs to slide out of the way of an incoming object. Damage to bladder, uterus, cervix and bowel will vary according to the violence of the entry and thrust. Damage to the perineum will be really bad with general body bruising around the waist.

Street rape is often of shorter duration than rape in a quieter place since fear of discovery is greater. It may be accompanied by a knife threat to subdue the victim faster without the need for using his own arms and legs in the overpowering.

The conundrum for the victim is that the more fight she puts up the worse her injuries will be. If there's really no way out and you haven't learnt any self-defence, talk. Talk and co-operate so he'll calm a tiny bit. If his urgency is quietened even a little and you intimate that you won't struggle because you don't want any damage done inside you, there's a chance he won't split the opening too badly. Use your own spittle, if your mouth hasn't completely dried with fear, and see if there's a second to put it on the vulva. Stand, lie or whatever, as still as you can under what are appalling circumstances. If two men are at it, the second may be easier because the ejaculate from the first will act as a lubricant.

When it's over go to the police immediately. Don't go home. Ring a door bell and ask whoever answers to dial 999. Stay on the doorstep unless an obviously reliable person answers. Remember all you can and fix descriptions in your mind for relating to the police. Don't wash, not even your hands. If you managed to scratch him, there could be valuable evidence under your nails of his blood group, tissue, hair and semen. These may also be on your clothes, underwear and perineal skin.

Only when the police doctor, usually a woman nowadays, has taken full swabs, tests and visual evidence should you bath and change, unless you are hospitalized.

Then put into action the Management of an Attack of Cystitis on page 159. Use plenty of cool bottled water down the perineum and inside the vagina to reduce the swelling. Bed rest will help a lot if you are not recommended for hospital, but even there, cooling air and cool water wash-downs will aid tissue healing enormously.

It may take several days, or a couple of weeks for soreness and bruising to go. During that time urinary infection or vaginal infection will start, if they are going to. More swabs and a urine test are essential to reveal any bacteria and to treat it accurately. A general broad-spectrum antibiotic may not be sensitive to the specific bacteria found in the samples, hence the accurate testing.

It may be well worthwhile to start talking straightaway

to a psychotherapist. Better to have the trauma out now than let it seep into your brain and cause years of anguish.

If you are desparately unfortunate enough to have serious internal organ damage, you may need a really first-class gynaecologist, urologist and proctologist (for the bowels) and tremendous courage and perseverance.

Sex for Handicapped People

In researching this section of the book I have come across several remarkable books on sex for disabled and chronically ill people, and I've included a small list for interest.

Paraplegics or tetraplegics, people with disabling diseases, people who have external bags instead of bowel or bladder are all still able in some way to make love. Account is taken of the disability, of course, but cuddling, handwork and a variety of penetration positions are perfectly possible.

That being so, all the usual preparations for healthy intercourse are still required. Scrupulous penile and perineal hygiene is mandatory. However, depending on the impaired mobility, it can be difficult or even impossible to go to a strange toilet set-up before intercourse. Where washing before intercourse may take able-bodied people twenty seconds or, conversely, be part of foreplay, so for the disabled person who has to be lifted on to a loo and washed, such activity can decidedly wreck the atmosphere of sexual arousal. When bowels are opened manually the disabled person performs careful hygiene then and tends to make that do for the day. All I am recommending here is that should urinary or vaginal problems tend to arise after sex then do revise and re-think your hygiene. In *Victims of Thrush and Cystitis*, there's a case history of a lady in a wheelchair. I revised her washing procedures to stop her bladder infections, and her bottle washing of the perineum after the daily bowel evacuation is worth a read if you are disabled and having a regular sex life.

It is quite incredible that internal organs all work despite the paralysis. Urine is still manufactured by the kidneys; blood still flows; digestion still breaks food into micro-particles and the uterus can still grow babies.

Contraception, therefore, needs discussion and experiment. Adverse reactions to contraceptives are just as likely to lead to urethritis, vaginitis and cystitis. Infection, although painless, can still result from intercourse and kidney involvement can become a real danger. Urinary retention harbours infection and encourages bladder bruising during intercourse.

I spoke to a married couple recently where the woman, aged fifty-five and her husband aged sixty-six are daily dealing with health troubles but still enjoying intercourse. Normal ageing is decreasing their libido and intercourse: once or twice a month is now their sexual pattern. Patricia has had multiple sclerosis for many years, had a hysterectomy in 1977 and had her tiresome, permanently infected bladder removed about five years ago. She now has a bag on her abdomen into which urine flows rather than down the ureters into the bladder. If her husband is really pressured into *his* preference over the years for her indwelling Foley catheter or now her external bag, he will say the bag. When they have intercourse, Patricia tucks the bag up under her nightie and, since the urostomy was performed, prefers to make love wearing clothing. Peter is quite wonderful about all of it and swears that because he loves her so much absolutely nothing impairs his sexual need and desire to show his love. Patricia's most comfortable sexual position is with a pillow under her buttocks. A bonus from the hysterectomy is that her once too-long vagina is now shortened and enables Peter to 'feel the top' and herself to enjoy it, too. Heavy abdominal scarring

146

plus the bag have, so Patricia says, made her feel less womanly, but Peter instantly counters this and warmly reassures her by, for instance, drawing attention to the relief from constant urinary infection caused by the Foley catheter and now non-existent, thanks to the bag. Their lovemaking is not impaired by bladder, kidney or vaginal infections.

A young girl, paralysed from her waist down at seventeen by a car crash, has now reached her thirty-fourth birthday. To be paralysed in her late teens at the time when most of us are first sexually active has to have been a mammoth blow. Jenny is still unmarried. Her parents, sister and a dog share a warm, loving home, and she has a variety of interests like sailing and lecturing to groups of nurses which keep her happy and active. Sexually, she had several men in her twenties but now such relationships are less frequent. Most men in her age group are married and the market supply has dwindled. Her increasing weight, she feels, makes her less attractive sexually but she looks well, has no obvious handicap except her wheel-chair and is a bright, jolly person to be with. She certainly isn't overweight.

Jenny's bowels are manually evacuated every other day and an external bag attached to her leg contains the constantly draining urine. Her bladder once had control but a period of stress and two lengthy holidays in the Seychelles dictated the preference for an indwelling Foley catheter. She has a permanent low-grade bladder infection from this, but it only occasionally requires antibiotics when it flares badly. There is no pain from the infection. Paralysed people run high temperatures and have smelly cloudy urine as an indication of infection.

To get into bed with a man means that Jenny must be lifted there. Her past partners have included handicapped and non-handicapped men. Some have been poor lovers, some good, some relationships have been lengthy, some short. Ask her what the requirements are for a good relationship if you are handicapped, and she says complete honesty, a lot of patient talking and a well-developed sense of humour. She has become well informed on literature for the disabled and has many books on sexuality which have been of great help in her sexual adventures. She admits that hygiene, although stringent under normal daily care of the perineum, takes a back seat in the efforts to gain interest, arousal and atmosphere once in a sexual situation.

Her spinal cord was crushed rather than broken in the car accident and so, vaginally, Jenny retains some feeling and loves penetration itself. From early missionary positions she and her boyfriends have experimented. Rear penetration when she is lying on her side is a favourite. Hugging, handwork and cuddling mean a lot to her – don't they to all of us? – and she would love to have a man to herself who would simply be there for the loving.

I recommend a book, *The Sexual Side of Handicap* published by Woodhead-Faulkner Ltd, Cambridge, and also *Sexual Problems and Their Management* published by Churchill Livingstone Medical Text, a branch of Longman's Ltd of London.

All these books have detailed dos and don'ts for happy intercourse, if you are in any way coping with handicap. The health aspects are manifold with much reference to infection of the bladder. It is pointless for my book here to try to be as effective as those specializing so closely in the field.

PART THREE

After Intercourse

In the Bathroom

It wasn't until July 1976 that I discovered the bottle-washing process which is so superb in preventing urinary infections and in reducing swelling after intercourse. It is fully described under 'Trichomonas' and in my other books, so here I want to add some extra tips, especially for use after intercourse.

A In a warm bathroom that contains both bath, basin and lavatory:

1 Fill up a mineral water bottle (not jug, glass or any other receptacle unless you're in an emergency setting) with *cool* water, not warm, and place it within easy reach of the lavatory. Wash your hands.

2 Sit on the lavatory, pass urine and then re-position the pelvis if necessary so that the legs are wide apart and the perineum attainable.

3 Slowly pour the *cool* water down the labia. Clean out the vagina with a long finger until all sexual liquid has gone and have a final pour over the whole perineum.

4 Pat dry with a soft flannel or guest towel until no moisture at all is left.

5 Drink something, tap water even, if there's nothing else available.

6 Go to bed to rest the perineum.

B In a warm house that has a separate lavatory from the bathroom:

1 Go to the bathroom first and fill two mineral water bottles with cool water. Wash your hands as well.

2 Carry the two bottles round the corner and into the lavatory.

3 Pass urine and then wash and proceed as above.

Do not use soap at all before or after intercourse.

The reason for the two bottles is in case one isn't quite enough so the second means that you can stay in the loo. If the bathroom has a loo as well, it's easier to refill the same bottle.

All of this takes thirty seconds only, when you've practiced it a couple of times. Missing it once can be enough to start cystitis, soreness or stinging. It's that important! Even if the house is cold *don't* stay in bed. Get up and do what must be done - the bed and he will warm you on your return.

If sex happens at another time, not night-time, the routine is just as normal *but* instead of going to sleep for eight hours, put on loose clothing. If you are staying indoors and relaxing keep a sexy colourful houserobe or caftan to wear for an hour or so. If you have to go to work or go shopping wear a longer skirt and loose underwear. No underwear at all would be even better, but do put on a clean petticoat or slip so that you sit on that if you sit down.

Resting for an hour or so is a big aid to cooling and contracting swollen perineal skin. Walking, jogging,

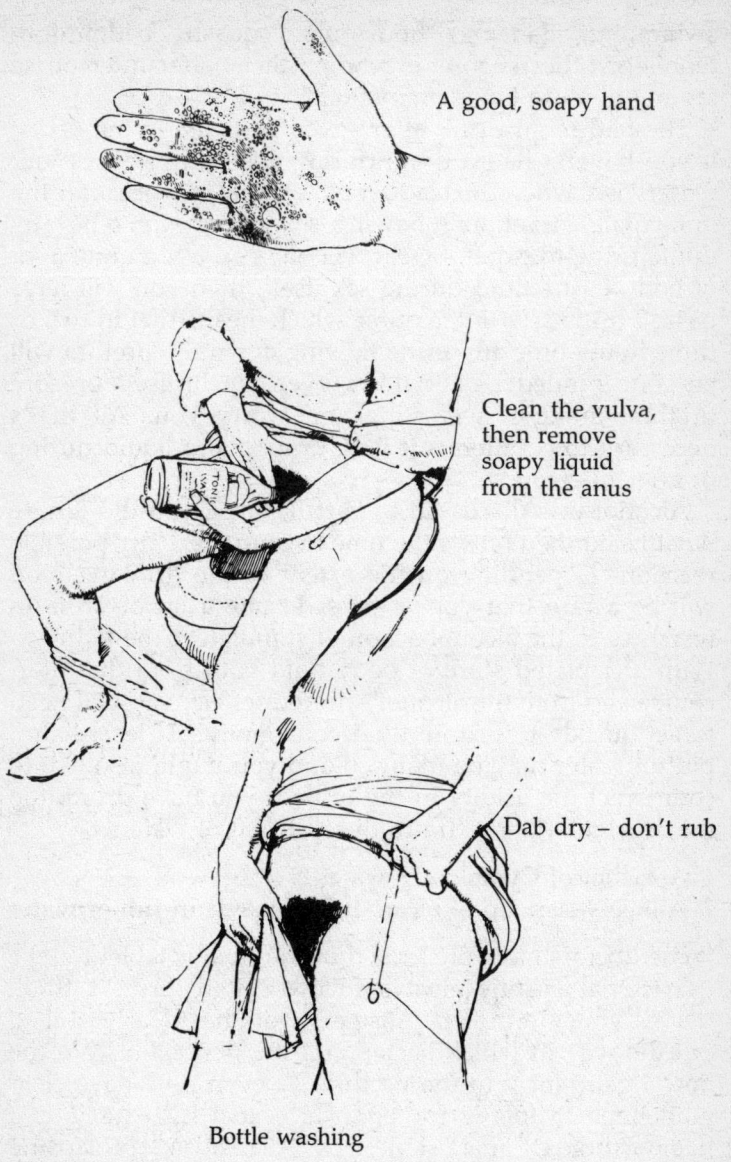

A good, soapy hand

Clean the vulva,
then remove
soapy liquid
from the anus

Dab dry – don't rub

Bottle washing

swimming, dancing, hoovering, squash, badminton, tennis or other such energetic pastimes after intercourse are not at all to be recommended.

The bathroom drink after sex is particularly important if you haven't had a drink during a lengthy sex session. Otherwise, when the bladder next wants to work after the immediate excretion following sex, there won't be any dilute urine to expel. Sweat will have excreted quite a lot of body tissue fluid during sex itself, then you will have passed urine after intercourse which means that in two or three hours time any urine flowing down the urethra will be concentrated. As it flows over the bruised or sore urethral lining it will sting and worry you. All that's necessary to counteract it is to drink bland liquid during or after intercourse.

Alcohol was discussed in Part II, but if you did ignore what I said then now's the time to counteract any possible reaction. Depending on the extent of the drinking, you will be aware that you've passed quite a lot of urine in response to the alcohol action of stimulating the kidneys. With a depleted store of body fluid both from the intercourse and from the alcohol's diuretic effect, you will need to act quickly to restore fluid equanimity. At least half a pint of water may be required and you might also like to counteract the acidity in the urine if you have drunk too much wine. Take, extra to the half-pint of water:

1 A sachet of Cymalon in water *or*
2 A level teaspoon of bicarbonate of soda in jam or water

Some doctors have prescribed one antibiotic tablet to take if bacterial cystitis always follows intercourse. I think that's dying out now because my work has clearly spelled out the way in which bacteria on the perineum from the bowel gain entry to the urethra. Women now have clear guidelines to follow for perineal sexual hygiene, but if haemorrhoids, anal skin tabs, diarrhoea, prolapsing urethral or vaginal lining are extra hazards then the hygiene will need backing up by appropriate medical care or surgical intervention.

If you are having a wonderfully lengthy sexual session and jelly as well as excitement is stopping you from being dry and giving up, it's quite possible to stop briefly for a visit to the loo to pass urine. Bottle wash after, instead of using loo paper. You kill the whole thing stone dead if you return to bed with a smell! No need to clean out the vagina, just pour a little water down the perineum, pat dry and return for further pleasure.

When contraceptive spermicidal cream or jelly needs to remain at the cervix for an hour or so, still bottle wash but don't clean out the vagina too high. Most of the sperm liquid will have been expelled down the vagina during muscular action involved in passing urine. Individual sperm of microscopic size may yet still be wriggling around the cervix hoping for a nifty swim up the cervical canal and into the uterus, so rather than become pregnant it's safer not to clean out too thoroughly.

Since cold water kills sperm, douching has been a much favoured method of contraception, especially in Catholic countries. A very attractive Greek lady I once knew had only ever used cold water or withdrawal and she had organized her one pregnancy well enough! Naturally some women are extremely fertile and such a douching with cold water could well not work at all. One of the awful dilemmas about fertility is that you don't know if you are fertile or infertile until an opportunity for a mistake or a planned pregnancy comes along. Maybe a cheap way to find out might make some scientist a wealthy man!

It's all very well spending time on the female when the male also needs corresponding hygiene. She won't like to make love to an unwashed partner and why should she take so much care if he doesn't pay similar attention to his own sexual cleanliness? It's not much fun after sex if the female has returned to bed smelling sweetly of Givenchy III, underarm talc and lavatorial loveliness if he's still flat out, sweaty, odorous, distinctly tacky and not about to rectify the matter. Remarks such as, 'I've put out a clean towel,' or 'The water's nice and warm,' or, 'That new soap is lovely,' ought to be taken seriously by any man and instantly recognized as a very sophisticated and cunning command to clean up!

All men should shower or bath each day. Men tend to sweat in their job, whether it's a desk or manual effort. That one act of washing each day is more effective at night so that bed-time sex has an automatic cleanliness. A shower after sex can be quick, just enough to get rid of the surface sweat and sexual odour. You can't possibly go to work next day smelling awful. If you are both into the occasional joys of bathing together before intercourse you need:

- A very warm bathroom, softly lit.
- Comfortably warm bathwater (hot water will make the vaginal opening swell up).
- A wide enough bath.
- Big warm towels.
- A nail brush.
- A smear of lubricating jelly inside the vagina already if penetration may be attempted.

You *don't* need:

- Hot water.
- Bath salts.
- Bath oil.
- Bubble baths.
- Bath foams.
- Deodorized or medicated soaps.
  Dettol in the bath–
  All of which can cause cystitis.

156

The beauty of the bottle washing lies in its effectiveness, its mobility of use and its nil cost. A bath or shower costs more than one or two bottles of tap water. Baths and showers, even in this age, aren't available the world over so travel with your bottle if necessary. Anywhere that water is scarce can often mean that it is contaminated as well. Filter the water first if you can or certainly boil it for several minutes. Then let it cool before bottling it and leaving it somewhere safe. You may remember to take a screw-on top to prevent airborne bacteria from entering.

If you are on a business trip, a short break or a longer holiday comes up, either take the bottle with you in a suitcase or ask for martini and soda at the hotel bar and hang on to the soda bottle. Chambermaids have whipped mine away before now so I'm careful to put it on a high shelf to indicate that I don't want it discarded.

This bottle is always clean inside and out simply because nothing and no-one else ever touches it. Firstly, it only ever contains water, and secondly, it is only ever held by freshly washed hands. If you have used a special cloth, sponge, or cotton wool up to now, stop doing so. A cloth or a sponge is easily infected and holds the bacteria in the dampness ready to go back on the perineum next time it's used. Cotton wool balls come expensive and you may eventually economize on liberal use of them – to say nothing of blocking up the lavatory.

Here again, I must emphasize that the bottle washing procedure (page 80) be followed each and every day of your life if you are prone to cystitis, urethritis and vaginitis and also if you aren't!

If your bowels work sporadically and not every day, this washing should still be done.

If you get diarrhoea, every bowel movement requires the full procedure.

If you pass a stool twice a day, employ the bottle washing each time.

If you have haemorrhoids, soap them and rinse extra thoroughly. Have them injected and have surgery if infections are regular.

I recommend *Understanding Cystitis – A Complete Self-help Guide*, published by Arrow Books, for more washing ideas, including bottle washing at work.

Counselling occasionally brings to light women who seem incapable of doing the bottle washing because they can't fathom out a way to deal with a *separate lavatory* situation.

- Keep *two* mineral water bottles by the basin.
- Keep the cloth for *drying* in the lavatory somewhere. Perhaps put up a hook or install a small cupboard so the cloth can't be mistaken for the one that cleans the lavatory seat.
- Walk through to the basin.
- Wash both hands well with soap and hot water. Rinse them.
- Fill the two bottles with warm water.
- Re soap one hand and soap the anus with it.
- Under a still-running hot tap, rinse that soapy hand.
- Pick up the two filled bottles and walk back into the separate lavatory with your soapy bottom.
- Sit down and wash the labia, clean out the vagina, ensure all soap has been rinsed away.
- After the last drops, pat dry the perineum very thoroughly with the drying cloth and pull up panties.
- Flush the lavatory and wipe the seat if necessary.
- Return the two empty mineral bottles to the bathroom ready for next time.

It's a simple enough system but some women can't seem to work it out.

An attack of cystitis starting after sex should be a thing

of the past once you have instituted the washing and anti-bruising tips. Should one start for that or any other reason:

- Have the urine checked properly, if it's streptococcus, staphylococcus, or E. Coli., it's still the hygiene.
- Negative urine can mean bruising, chemical or allergic reaction, contraceptive trouble etc.
- Soreness and twingeing can mean vaginal discharge of any sort affecting both vagina and urethra.

Management of an Attack of Cystitis

1. Take a urine sample. Store it in the fridge, but try to get it to a doctor or lab, fast. Ask for the result when it comes through.
2. Drink half a pint of water straight away, and take three strong painkillers with it.
3. Make two hot water bottles, one for the back and one in a towel for between your legs.
4. Take one level teaspoon of bicarbonate of soda/Effercitrate/mis. pot. cit./Cymalon to alkalanise the acidity and reduce the burning.
5. Stay near a lavatory and rest.

Repeat the half-pint of water every twenty minutes for three hours.
Repeat the alkalanizing twice more in three hours.
Repeat painkillers as the packet instructs.
Read *Understanding Cystitis – A Complete Self-help Guide* for greater detail.
Re-read the book, have a gynaecological examination or come for counselling.

Case Histories

The kinds of sexual cystitis that women bring to me in counselling are quite varied, and to end the third part of the book I've written up some case histories for your interest. If you feel that you have some aspect of sexual cystitis not covered in this book that I may like to include in a future update, please write to me c/o the publishers and enclose an SAE if you would like my comments. Counselling, if you are completely stuck, is very valuable.

I also run short courses of three classes both in cystitis and candida. For further details please send an SAE to my publishers.

Cynthia Gale

Cynthia Gale came referred to me from a urologist. She has had cystitis with kidney complications and vaginal thrush since she was eighteen. Now aged twenty-four, numerous visits to various hospitals in London have persuaded her that there is nothing medically wrong, but that, despite negative results, she still has chronic cystitis with flare-ups of pyelitis. Pyelitis is inflammation and infection of the kidneys. Between 1985–1986 she has been hospitalized five times with high temperatures, vomiting and abnormal blood cell counts in her burning urine.

According to all the urine tests ever taken by various laboratories there is no significant bacteria in the samples, nor has infection been proven in the kidneys. Despite this, antibiotics have been administered and thrush has become the third problem.

Cynthia is a computer programmer trainer. Although, strictly speaking, her job is nine to five each day, it is more often seven in the morning until nine at night and includes a great deal of travelling. The large company for which she works specializes in providing computer trainers and there are four, including Cynthia, in her group who teach mostly in the north west of the country. One week she will sit solidly in front of a VDU screen in deep concentration and moving only for lunch; the next week she will take that week's work on tour and teach it to the people who will take over their firm's computer programming or training. The stress and concentration levels are extremely high – one wrong button pressed and a week's work is wrecked. On tour she stays with the other three members of her group in hotels, so she has company and a good expenses-paid dinner with wine each night.

Robin is thirty-six years old and an accountant. He met Cynthia fifteen months ago and they soon became sexually involved. Six months ago they began to stay for long periods in each other's flats and one month ago Cynthia moved into Robin's flat. They now live together and are very happy.

Neither have time for hobbies, sport or real relaxation. From Friday night through to Sunday they catch up on washing, ironing, shopping, sex and seeing friends. Alcohol features throughout the weekend with Cynthia particularly into white wine and gin and tonic. All weekend, except for dining out, both wear casual clothes: trousers or jeans with attractive tops. Indeed Cynthia wore blue corded trousers and a checked sweater for her visit to me.

She has never read any of my books.

Symptoms

Cystitis attacks take the form of frequency in passing urine, burning urine and low pubic pain. Often she has a high temperature, vomiting, malaise and may even go straight there without urethral involvement. Not every sex session produces cystitis or twingeing but most do. Amounts of urine passed at the beginning of attacks are small and dark, but since doctors told her to drink more on the first twinges, urine is now paler. She is always tired and sometimes feels bloated. Since thrush accompanies all

162

courses of antibiotics she now receives anti-fungal treatment with the antibiotics.

General Health

Apart from having her wisdom teeth out and a toe straightened under anaesthetic there have been no other operations at all.

Other than the health matters for which she visited me, there are no major problems. She gets occasional migraines, night leg aches and crampy feelings. Cynthia, although underweight, looks well and is a very alert person.

Urological Investigations

Mid-stream urine tests	All negative of bacteria but dark with abnormal red/white cell results.
Intra-venous pyelogram (kidney X-ray)	Reports no abnormalities, 1986.
Cystoscopy	Not done.
Ultra scan of bladder and kidneys	No abnormality. Plenty of hospitalization for pyelitis and specialist discussion.

Gynaecological History

Apart from Family Planning visits for pap smears and cap fittings, Cynthia has not been carefully scrutinized. Her periods began aged sixteen years with little discomfort or blood loss. She uses Tampax and occasionally sanitary towels.

Contraceptive History

From eighteen to twenty years old the Pill was taken. From twenty to twenty-two years old, Cynthia used the cap with its accompanying spermicidal foams and jellies. Much cystitis occured in this two-year period. Her next

163

boyfriend had no objections to the sheath and for their year-long relationship this form of contraception was used on the limited occasions when sex took place. Because the incidence of intercourse rose once Robin came into her life, Cynthia went on the mini-pill Norgeston and has remained on it for fifteen months.

Hygiene

On Friday evenings both Cynthia and Robin shower. Cynthia passes a stool in the mornings, but doesn't wash afterwards. After the evening shower (she used to bath until moving in with Robin a month ago, but he has a super new shower unit and she enjoys using it) they both make love. After intercourse she rushes off to the bathroom, passes urine and rushes back to bed without washing because the house is too cold. Robin turns the heating off before going to bed.

Intercourse

There is sometimes a session on a midweek night, but mostly, due to a heavy working week, sex occurs several times over each weekend. Friday night is the first, possibly Saturday morning, possibly Saturday evening or Sunday morning dependent sometimes on how tiddly Robin is by Saturday night! Sometimes Sunday evening may find a top-up session but it is rare. Overall they make love between three and five times in any seven-day period.

The amount of time spent in penetrative sex varies from half a hour to an hour, all dependent on how tired generally they both feel from the working week. Cystitis and pyelitis can arise from lengthy sessions or short highly energetic ones and usually start off as soreness. This soreness extends over a couple of days into real trouble. Real trouble means anxiety, tension, fear, pain, drugs, doctors, hospital, off work, off sex.

A telling phrase Cynthia used in counselling was, 'The

more enjoyable the sex, the more likely I am to start cystitis.'

Being young and in love, Cynthia is lubricating well. Her vagina is very wet when she's aroused and there is no discomfort either on penetration or during intercourse itself. An excellent sign. Positions are variable and enjoyable and none appear to hurt, but she may come to rethink this. Of the six men with whom she has had intercourse since she was eighteen, Robin and the first man, Simon, appear to have coincided with the worst sex/cystitis patterns. Neither man is circumcised.

Liquid Intake

Fairly satisfactory. Cynthia drinks one pint of water each morning and at lunchtime because the doctors have advised this to protect the kidneys. She voids (empties) a lot which is just as important as the intake, and I found that reasonably satisfactory too. What I didn't like was the intake of alcohol. She's not read any of my work, on the link between alcohol and sex.

Diet

Cynthia's diet is a mixture. That's good. She eats well and does so to maintain energy at work. Lunch is always taken and she has good dinners either at home with Robin or with her group in hotels on tour. Soft fruit or citrus fruits are absent, though she may eat an occasional apple. At home she often makes curries but doesn't include all the spices and makes them very mild. About once a fortnight she and Robin will eat a curry out. She doesn't take pepper.

Clothing

At work it's always dresses or skirts and tops. At weekends its always trousers or jeans unless on a special outing. Underwear is stockings, suspender and cotton undies.

Bad Habit

Long soaky hot baths until one month ago when Robin's shower took over.

Weight

At eight stone four pounds and five foot five inches tall, she is small-boned and well-proportioned. When she stands up, her trousers are loose across the pubic bone area but tight underneath. Cynthia can reach nine stone at times like Christmas, but hates herself at that weight and promptly diets down again.

Ideas and Suggestions

If you read *Victims of Thrush and Cystitis* published by Arrow, you will see how I set about counselling. During counselling I have, at one side of me, two pieces of paper, separated by carbon, on which I write bright ideas in a list as they occur to me. I enlarge on these in later discussion, and the patient takes the top copy home with her. That way we both know where we stand and reference can be made, if necessary, in later phone calls. So, as the ideas came during Cynthia's session with me here they are:

1 Go to eight stone twelve pounds with Christmas coming up to help. Thin skin bruises.
2 Don't use Tampax.
3 Take mineral supplements.
4 Highly sensitive metabolism and skin.
5 The Dutch cap bruises the cervix when pummelled during intercourse.
6 Jelly and foam spermicides can irritate the cervix and vagina.

7 Hygiene necessary after sex.

8 No more trousers or jeans. The seam squashes the vulva. Culottes are OK.

9 Alcohol and sex together spell *trouble*. Limit and balance alcohol if sex is likely.

10 After sex – no underwear. Rest up. Skin needs to cool and contract.

11 Alcohol just by itself can cause cystitis or pyelitis. Dehydration by alcohol removes liquid which kidneys need. Excess uric acid, undiluted, causes burning urine.

12 Bicarbonate of soda/cymalon/mis.pot.cit./Effercitrate will all help to alkalinize burning urine by counteracting acidity.

13 Look at the Management of an Attack of Cystitis on page 159.

14 Turn the heating off *after* intercourse. Then you can be warm whilst washing.

15 After sex, pass urine and then pour cool water down the perineum, hooking out all sexual liquids. Pat absolutely dry.

16 Always have a glass of water after sex. Go and rest, don't put on any clothing so that air can cool and heal the swollen vulva.

17 Space the sex sessions.

18 Use lubricating jelly even though you're wet. It will give extra padding to your thin vagina and sensitive bladder, thus absorbing the thrust shocks.

19 Cut out the curries.

My comments

I chose the weight of eight stone twelve pounds to stop short of Cynthia's instinctive abhorrence of being nine stone! She has agreed to put on weight following my revelations on thin skin not absorbing penile thrusting. For now, and possibly the future as well, the lubricating jelly will act as a shock absorber. Cynthia's own vaginal wetness is insufficient padding when faced with the pelvic muscle thinness.

Tampons are drying and chemicals are used in the production both of the cotton wool and the applicator. Use them sparingly if ever.

When long-term illness or debilitating drugs begin to feature, then the body must be helped to cope by introducing mineral supplements. A lot of work is being done now on zinc deficiency in women. Take 'Zinc with Minerals' tablets regularly. Night cramping, tiredness, poor sleeping plus migraines, headaches and other symptoms can disappear magically with magnesium B.13 supplement. Iron, we all know, is a useful and long-used mineral supplement for menstruating women. You may also be in need of others like chromium, for instance. Have a mineral assessment made from laboratory analysis of your hair and sweat. Many allergic (highly sensitive) people have mineral deficiencies – are you one of them?

Cynthia had already seen the effects of the cap and its accompanying spermicidal foams and creams for herself. She has decided never to use this contraceptive method again.

The seam of jeans or tight trousers causes vulval pressure. If you press your finger on to a hard surface like a table for five minutes it will become white and indented at the point of contact. When the blood returns, the end of the finger will swell a little. This same process will occur on the uretheral and vaginal openings if you jam a seam up them! Have intercourse afterwards and you add swelling skin to already swollen skin! The trouble is twofold because inside jeans or trousers, most women wear panties. These are washed in the machine using some kind of soap or biological powder. You wouldn't dream of putting that powder on your tongue – why force it into the urethral and vaginal openings?

Don't wear tights under trousers. Air cannot circulate and cool the skin. Cynthia doesn't do this but it's worth a mention for those who do. I recommend no clothing on the perineum at all if you are recovering from a session of intercourse. If you're prone to thrush generally or cystitis from sexual bruising don't wear underwear at home. Just wear a longer skirt, and rest for an hour.

Alcohol dries out all body cell liquid *everywhere*, not just the mouth! The kidneys manufacture more urine and uric acid because the alcohol has 'excited' them, and when the bladder has excreted most of it the mouth is the first place to display the drying up process. The vagina and bladder are just two more parts of the body to dry up. Less cell liquid means less tissue and muscle padding to absorb the penile thrusting. Alcohol must be severely restricted if sex is to be unaffected. Balance its effect with a couple of glasses of water, not canned, sweetened drinks because of thrush-loving sugar.

Upstairs in my bathroom, I took Cynthia through the bottle-washing process after sex. This is no problem, but she knows now to keep the central heating on until after sex so that she won't feel cold. It's not that the bottle process is lengthy, but if you don't fancy the cold bathroom you'll be put off going into it!

Drink a glass of water after the washing so that the next time you pass urine it won't be dark and stingy. Energetic sex makes you sweat and the passing of urine after sex, which is mandatory, does mean that those lost body liquids must be replaced. Just drink.

Spacing sex makes sense in terms of reducing swelling. The working week puts a heavy emphasis on weekend sex, so there's less chance for cervical, vaginal, vulval, and perineal skin to contract and cool. The bladder and urethra, too, need time to relax. This may actually be a big factor in the attack.

I don't know how much effect the curries are having.

Her symptoms aren't screaming to my instincts that the curries are a cause. However, not having read anything on cystitis before seeing me, Cynthia may not have had her own ideas fully in order. Perhaps occasional twingeing and soreness is happening due to mild curry and lager on a Saturday, but with such regular sex this may be masking the effect of the curry. The curries are best left alone for a while until my self-help sex suggestions have been implemented.

In conjunction with self-help I may suggest a thorough gynaecological survey, but nothing at the moment suggests any vaginal disease or abnormality. Cynthia is lubricating well and despite the alcohol intake, intercourse is free from any discomfort. Vaginal thrush corresponds to antibiotics and she does not get it at other times, although she may have low-grade body candida which could be invading the trigone. I think this is unlikely because she would be telling me other symptoms which I know through experience to be more relevant.

Cynthia has bought *Understanding Cystitis A Complete Self-help Guide* and pronouces it amazing. After six years of trouble with a capital T she may now be on the right road at last and two months will show us the result.

Telephone Follow Up – 31 December

Cynthia rang with some bad, some good news. The bad news is that over the Christmas period two minor attacks of cystitis began. Both were on a Sunday when the laboratories were shut and so she didn't bother to take a urine sample. With my book and its procedures now being read, absorbed and practiced, she aborted both attacks herself with the 'Management of an Attack' procedure within four hours. No symptoms hung about so she didn't bother to phone me or the doctor. This new skill thrilled her particularly because she knew that she had prevented the cystitis from turning into pyelitis with all its abundant miseries. The bad news of more cystitis turned into good news, providing her with the opportunity to try out a procedure that will always bring relief from pain and fear.

Obviously, though, the two further attacks means more detailed thought on the reason or reasons behind them. Both began after the weekend's sex session, so we look still to sex as the cause, but what in the sex is specifically encouraging the cystitis? Also, without urine tests we don't know whether bacteria were there or not.

A major revelation was made by Cynthia on relating a phone call from her doctor. Very casually he announced that there had in fact been a lot of mid-stream urine specimens in the past that had been positive. Cynthia was furious with him, more so because he had known that she was coming to see me and that I had asked to be informed of urine results. Only after our counselling session had he checked her notes, revised his and telephoned the news to her.

So now we have both factors of sexual cystitis – bacterial cystitis *and* non-bacterial cystitis. Thank goodness I had gone thoroughly into the bottle-washing procedure anyway!

Cynthia is bottle washing now with great care and had done so over Christmas. Were those two attacks just the result of a traumatized vagina and urethra? We will never know because there were no urine tests.

However, I had a request. It was that she and Robin have no weekend intercourse for six weeks, so that urine samples could be taken to a laboratory on a weekday. I also stipulated the nights on which intercourse should take place: Monday and Wednesday. This spaces the sex, enabling the vagina to recover on Tuesday and Thursday, it also means possibly that alcohol will be further restricted since they both have to be fit for work the next day!

More good news was that, thanks to Christmas, she has begun to put on the weight I suggested and was past eight stone nine pounds and towards the eight stone twelve pounds that I would like. We may still need one of my good gynaecologists to look up her vagina.

13 February

Cynthia rang out of the blue just before I had mentally clocked up the six weeks in which I wanted the spaced sex.

At first, I didn't really remember her. This was specifically because the voice tone level didn't sound like hers, it sounded higher, maybe a tone and a half by my musical ear. I told her about this after our chat and suggested that it might be because her mind had lightened with the good news and the strong prospect of having conquered her own brand of cystitis.

During those six weeks of specifically spaced intercourse there had not even been one twinge of trouble! I could hear the excitement in her voice. So no lab tests on urine samples had been needed and intercourse on the Monday and Wednesday had been extended to include one at the weekend as well.

I asked her what *she* felt were the prime reasons for the release from symptoms and she listed first:

Washing after passing a stool, then

Evenly spaced sex.

The beautiful simplicity of correct, timely washing with the bottle is absolutely marvellous and Cynthia is in no doubt as to its value. She also understands the need for the vagina to recover from intercourse and this, too, is a lifetime's valuable lesson. Alcohol is now restricted and a better weight has been attained. At eight stone twelve pounds, extra padding all over the body, including the pelvic region, helps the vagina to absorb penile thrusting and not be so badly shocked by it.

Cynthia is thrilled and so am I. I always am. It's not the first and it won't be the last, but my thrill for each woman who gets free from cystitis is simply as though it were for myself. Remember her case history: sexual cystitis used to put her in hospital with kidney complications. No doctor and no drugs stopped her attacks – prevention did.

Linda Willett

Linda Willett is twenty-eight years old and a bright, energetic graphics designer. Being self-employed she can work in any market area requiring design, but so far finds most of her employment in the world of women's magazines, books and classical music publishers. She spent four years training at the Canterbury College of Design and has never looked back. Constant work means that she must live in London and she shares a flat with three other women.

Until February 1986 she had one boyfriend, Mike, for seven years but that ended when Steven arrived in her life at a Christmas party. Steven is also a graphics designer which was probably one reason why they hit it off from the start. She spends most weekends with Steven in his flat but during the week she goes back to the flat-share. The weekend pattern is one of food, drink, sex, odd jobs and relaxation.

Symptoms

Nasty attacks of cystitis always following intercourse since 1979. Attacks comprise pain, frequency in passing urine and bleeding, and start twenty-four to thirty-six hours after sex. Antibiotics have always been used and in turn have caused a lot of vagina and body candida which, too, has needed treatment. Irritation around the anal orifice worsens or starts during the week before a period and this has been happening since 1981. Between January and August, Linda has had four bad attacks of cystitis. She has no headaches or back aches and apart from thrush has no other bladder or vaginal difficulties.

Urological Investigations

Mid-stream urine tests .	Lots, which always show infection.
Intra-venous pyelogram	One which was negative.
Cystoscopy	None.

Gynaecological History

Her *periods* began when she was aged thirteen and are trouble free. She has had no gynaecological operations and has never been pregnant.

Contraceptive History

The need for this began in 1979 when Linda met Mike. The microgynon contraceptive Pill was chosen for two years until it was stopped because of thrush. From then on, condoms or the diaphragm (cap) were used but all cystitis attacks between January and August have occurred when the cap was employed.

General Health

Good.

Bowels

Also good. She usually passes a stool at work and therefore has not washed afterwards, nor does she at any other time.

Hygiene

Poorly average. No hygiene after a stool or after sex. Linda and Steven do bath together before sex but she doesn't wash her perineal area because she feels too awkward about doing so in front of him. The house-share lavatory is only cleaned once a week and so is Steven's. Steven is not circumcised. She likes long hot baths.

Alcohol

Linda likes a drink but has already realized that alcohol is bad for women prone to cystitis.

Diet

Not too bad but has a regular intake of carbohydrates like rice and potatoes and sugar. Canned drinks and coffee are snatched at work.

Bedding

She has half-poly, half-cotton sheets and blankets.

Work Conditions

Linda's job keeps her sitting down, usually on the edge of a hard chair so that she can draw, paint or design.

Clothing

She wears trousers and tights.

Ideas and Suggestions

1 Baths! get in – get out! They are hot and wet.
2 Nystatin oral anti-fungal tablets should always be taken with any course of antibiotics if you are thrush/monilia prone.
3 Reduce or cut the carbohydrate and sugar input.
4 Eat three tablespoons of live yoghurt before each meal in the week before a period. Insert lactic acid pessaries or Aci Jel jelly into the vagina to counteract the alkalinity of the vagina and arrival of thrush/monilia.
5 Always ask for the urine test result.
6 Don't use the cap for contraception again.
7 Hygiene must improve. Use the bottle washing. In your case at work, at Steven's flat, at the flat-share. Have three bottles, three wash cloths for drying, three

bars of good soap, three toilet bags, three kitchen towel rolls.

8 Recap: Use *warm* water and soap after passing a stool at work or at home.

Use *cool* water, no soap, after sex.

9 No canned drinks or sugar.

10 Beware of bedding that produces a sweaty or sticky bed and therefore an overheated body which promotes thrush/monilia.

11 Avoid intercourse before a period until thrush is controlled. Not only may Steven catch it, but the heat generated in sex will help thrush.

12 Before using Steven's loo or the flat-share loo, clean it! Keep a cloth and cleanser and don't forget the flush handle!

13 It is very important for Steven to retract and wash under the foreskin. Show him this list if you feel too shy about directly telling him.

14 Following penetration it helps to keep still for thirty seconds or more so that the vagina can relax open and acclimatize to the introduction of the penis.

15 At work vary the time you sit on the chair. Stand at regular intervals.

16 Go without underwear at home. Wear skirts to work and stockings and suspenders, not tights. One pair of pure cotton panties is fine but no trousers or jeans.

17 The perineum must be allowed air at all times so also cut the pubic hair every five to six weeks, with scissors, to half an inch.

Linda never had cystitis or thrush before she began to have intercourse. This very simple but honest fact makes her a victim of sexual cystitis. Vaginal thrush/Monilia came a fast second in her trouble because the antibiotics cleared out her gut defences and enabled fungus to infiltrate the lining of the wet mucous areas of her body, including the vagina.

The correct order of sorting out the muddle is finding the reason/s associated with sexual intercourse which are causing the cystitis so that, without any more cystitis, there will be no need for antibiotics.

Obviously the cap contraceptive was an easy thing to stop straight away so other contraceptives have to be discussed. We talked around all sorts and Linda also agreed to have a chat to her doctor.

All the points about thrush became relevant and we spent some time on this because thrush can also cause cystitis. It make senses to work at reducing the yeast by prevention so it would be less likely to cause an odd attack of cystitis that would frustrate careful elimination work on other points.

Apart from not having had cystitis before starting intercourse, the second great clue to the cause of attacks comes from the urine samples. They are all positive. Although the bacteria are not named, and we shouldn't make an assumption, we are left with the probability that bowel bacteria of some sort are in the urine samples. This is backed up by the knowledge that Linda never washes after a stool nor is any sexual hygiene practised.

Before Linda can do the bottle washing in peace, several social situations have to be understood and dealt with. Firstly, she has three distinct buildings in whose lavatories she is likely to have a bowel movement: work, Steven's flat and the flat-share with the three other girls. Secondly, these three places don't all have the ideal bathroom arrangement of basin, lavatory and bath in the one room. So we have to design one system that will allow her to wash properly in any of the buildings at any time.

I decided that the simplest way was to keep a set of every item required in the bottle-washing routine at each building so it was always there for use even if Linda wasn't. To keep each set clean and private, I suggested a cheap but sizeable toiletry bag to hold everything.

The shopping list therefore comprised:

three sizeable toiletry/cosmetic bags.
three mineral or soda water bottles (each to fit a toiletry bag).
three wash cloths or guest towels.
three bars of a pure soap.
one tube of lubricating jelly (to be kept at Steven's flat for sex).
three kitchen paper towel rolls.

The kitchen towel roll is an additional item because the work-place toilets, and those in the two flats, have no basin in with the lavatory. By tearing off a couple of sheets, moistening and soaping them *before* going into the lavatory cubicle or the separate lavatory in the flats, Linda will be able to soap her back passage when ready and stay in the cubicle.

The mineral or soda water bottle is also filled before entering the cubicle or separate lavatory and placed on a shelf or on the floor on another sheet of the kitchen roll to avoid contact with the floor itself. The filled bottle of very warm water is also ready to use as required.

Because of the atrocious bathroom cleaning both at Steven's and the flat-share, I insisted that Linda installed her own lavatory cleanser and cloth using them before she sat on the seat! At work I asked her to line the lavatory seat with toilet tissue or kitchen roll and to use a single sheet over the flush handle when she pulled it.

It's true that in some circumstances the kitchen towel roll could also be used for drying the perineum after washing, but I'm not at all sure that minute bits of paper won't be left behind on the skin so I'd feel safer using the small linen guest towel or a flannel.

So much for the hygiene. I wanted Linda to reduce her

alcohol intake at the weekends when sexual activity was likely. Sex plus alcohol is no good! So – stop the alcohol (or drastically reduce it) and drink water during lengthy sex if you feel like it. But always after it when you've finished in the bathroom.

After a couple of hours' counselling, Linda departed. I told her to telephone me whenever necessary for discussion because she had had a lot to digest and might not have some ideas quite straight enough. Being intelligent she will doubtless manage and we'll wait and see how she gets on.

Follow Up

Five months later, on reaching this section of *Sexual Cystitis*, I picked up the telephone and rang for a report. Linda's voice sounded delighted to hear me and said that on her desk was a written but unposted letter to tell me how well she had been and that despite plenty of sex there had only been one cystitis attack. This was an all-time record and she was thrilled. She had been very thorough in the revision of her lifestyle and had not cut any corners.

She was also amazed to hear me because a week previously, after returning to Steven from the two-week Christmas break with her family in the country, they had made up for the lack of Christmas sex! This involved four or five acts of intercourse in twenty-four to thirty-six hours and cystitis began! The attack began on a Sunday and, with no doctor or lab open for testing, she had succumbed in fright to taking antibiotics left over in the medicine chest.

I pointed out that:

1 This attack may not have involved bacteria.
2 It might only have been bruising and inflammation.

179

3 It might have been brought on by vaginal thrush from Christmas chocolates and wines.

4 If points one and three were true, then antibiotics were not necessary and would prolong or worsen any vaginal thrush.

5 If such circumstances happen again *don't* take antibiotics until *after* a urine test and vaginal swab have been taken on the Monday morning. Until the Monday morning use 'Management of Attack' to protect the kidneys and limit discomfort in the bladder and urethra.

She then realized she'd made a mistake in taking the antibiotics and having too much sex, but for this attack it's too late except, maybe, to have a swab for thrush taken.

Linda has recently moved to a new flat which she shares with one friend only. The new flat has the perfect bathroom – basin, lavatory and bath in one room. So she has asked my permission to stop using the soapy kitchen towel sheets and move on to the perfect bottle-washing routine of soaping a hand and using that to clean the anal orifice. This impressed me greatly and was positive proof that she fully understood what I had taught her.

Despite the setback, her spirits were unaffected because she had thought the post-Christmas attack through and *learnt* from it. Next time she and Steven meet up after being apart they will take care to space the sex and reduce trauma.

I also chatted about the long-term prospects for a cystitis victim like herself. Having triumphed over the sex side she may (or may not) find it coming at later times like those mentioned on the first page of this book but these, too, can be overcome. My work has also reduced the sheer fear of cystitis which is often overwhelming for so many women. Cystitis is beatable, regard it as an enemy which can be tactically beaten with the right weapons.

Jane Johnson

Jane Johnson has been a fan of mine apparently for many years and had the earliest edition of my book, *Understanding Cystitis* first published in 1972. In that book there was only one chapter on self-help. Obviously in view of what I have researched and written since then, that humble chapter was inadequate – historical in its encouragement to women to adopt specific self-help procedures, but still inadequate. She hadn't updated her bookshelf with my own advancing knowledge and so, when she arrived in a desperate state for counselling in July 1986, there was much said that was new to her.

Jane is now forty years old, vivacious, good looking, but worried and distressed. Her sexual history, going back to 1968, is packed with awful sadness caused by poor sexual health. Both the bladder and vagina have ruled her life and diminished all personal fulfilment and aspiration. Her two children, John and Luke, are eleven and four respectively, and have come from two past relationships. Other than looking after their needs she just about copes with part-time teaching in one of England's universities. In trying to overcome her troubles she seems keen on taking holidays in Europe, but these are invariably at the best miserable, and at the worst, wrecked to the point of returning home.

She and her first husband, Tim, were virgins when they married aged twenty-two years old. Neither had experienced another partner and were very much in love. From day one of this union their marriage was doomed to pain, frequency in passing urine, doctors, drugs and restricted intercourse between constant attacks of cystitis – much like my own, except that Jane directly attributes her divorce to cystitis – and my marriage survived that. Tim was grossly inexpert at making love. He had, by standards she learned later, an enormous penis which was uncircumcised and which penetrated her without any foreplay or easing in. He ejaculated within the first two or three minutes of frantic thrusting. She had little enjoyment and much following distress. In those seven years, 1968–1975, my work was first absent and then only just beginning, which is why, too late, she found my first book. She cried with the relief on reading about my own experiences and set about some self-help. Some minor improvements began but because of the combination of her poor hygiene and Tim's poor behaviour in bed she was still swamped with fear and creased up by painful bladder infections. After seven years she and Tim separated and divorced. They had had no children.

It is now eighteen years since her first marriage, and this woman is still moved to tears as she recounts her great love for the man with whom she chose to spend her life, and whom, because of cystitis, she was denied.

After her divorce Chris came on the scene and was an instinctively better lover. There was much foreplay between them and he would spend twenty minutes or more inside her before a good ejaculation. Jane by now, from my first book, knew to get up after sex and pass urine. Sometimes she washed but never by the bottle-washing method, because it hadn't been discovered. Any washing might have been with a wet cloth or by sitting in the bath. Cystitis lessened but her time with Chris still saw several attacks of cystitis followed by thrush from the antibiotics.

When this relationship ended, Owen came along. They fell in love and remained together for four years, though did not marry. Jane's first child, John, was fathered by Owen who, again, had a large penis. An inexperienced lover, he nevertheless caught on quite well to Jane's whispered ideas and needs, and his earlier fast ejaculations became more controlled as he tried to pleasure her and help her avoid attacks of cystitis. These still occurred but not with such frequency.

Perry helped pick up the pieces of the ending of her relationship with Owen and was an instant thrill. He showed her for a year what a really skilled lover can do. Although large, he so played her that not once in a year did Jane have cystitis and, according to Jane, they made love by night and by day. It was and remains her most loved and successful 'normal' year ever.

Guy became Jane's second husband. There was plenty of foreplay and he was good in all bed respects. He is also the father of little Luke. Cystitis was virtually absent in their two-year marriage, for which Jane was heartily thankful. She now numbered three years of good sexual health.

After the failure of marriage number two for reasons other than poor health, Jane and Patrick became lovers from 1984, bringing the story up to date. Patrick is so-so in bed. His penis is the smallest one of all the five previous partners and with only a modicum of foreplay, little invention and no flair, he ejaculates about five minutes after penetration. Cystitis has rampaged through Jane from day one with Patrick and it's a miracle that he is still with her. They don't live together but he often stays at her home and they holiday together.

In counselling Jane was persuaded to mark her men out of ten for their sexual expertise:

Tim – 3
Chris – 8
Owen – 5
Perry – 10
Guy – 8
Patrick – 6

So, on an overcast summer day, Jane sat before me not only to recount her sadness on losing Tim but also to ask my help in sorting her out thoroughly.

Symptoms

Attacks of cystitis since the age of twenty-two always following sex. Attacks contain fever, back ache, headache, pain on passing urine, frequency in passing urine, bleeding. Additionally there is a vaginal discharge and a sore perineum. Vaginal thrush usually comes after any antibiotics.

Urological Investigations

Mid-stream urine samples have been taken for many years, but the GP doesn't bother to test – he just doles out antibiotics. Intra-venous Pyelogram: Never. Cystoscopy and cautery in the early 1970s.

Children

John, 1976 Forceps delivery, epidural anaesthetic, stitches.

Luke, 1983 Epidural anaesthetic, stitches.

Contraceptive History

Since Jane's first marriage, the major contraceptive has been the diaphragm (cap) used with spermicidal jelly. There was one year when three different types of Pill were tried but all types produced unwelcome side effects and further attempts were abandoned.

Intercourse

This has varied as per the explanations of the men. Jane is too sore now to tolerate any penetration though penetration itself doesn't hurt, but over several years she has felt more and more sore during sex. Sometimes it's all right, but not always. Intercourse mostly takes place at night. Cystitis will either start the next day or three days later. Rear penetration produces discomfort.

Hygiene

Jane never washes after passing a stool. From my books she has learnt to get up and pass urine after sex but this has only been for ten years. For the whole of her first marriage she didn't pass urine or wash. Even now she sometimes can't be bothered and her last attack was probably neglect. She showers or baths when she likes.

Liquid Intake and Diet

Reasonably all-round except that she says she knows that her system is acid and so she restricts her fruit intake. Coffee is not drunk at all. Food in general is of good quality meat and vegetables.

Ideas and Suggestions

1 A really good gynaecologist. I gave her a referral.
2 During and after all antibiotics, ask for (insist on!) Nystatin oral tablets as thrush prevention.
3 a You must use lubricating jelly before and during intercourse.
  b Avoid rear entry since it seems to increase discomfort.
  c Always use the bottle-washing process after sex. The water should be cool and all sexual liquids must be hooked out from the vagina whilst pouring. No soap is needed on the anus. The cool water eases the swelling.
  d Don't use the cap and spermicidal cream. Try the sponge.
  e For now, though hopefully not after seeing the gynaecologist, take one or two painkillers after sex to calm bladder nerve endings. Drink water after intercourse.

5 Bottle wash as demonstrated and as written in this book after every bowel movement.
6 If another attack starts:
   a Take and store a urine sample. Get it to the doctor.
   b Drink close to a pint of water immediately on the first twinges.
   c Take three strong painkillers.
   d Take one level teaspoon of bicarbonate of soda in water or jam.
   e Ring the gynaecologist again and make an urgent appointment for a urine test and swabs.
7 The reason for the attacks, judging by their timing – starting after intercourse – appears to be infection.

My Comments

We commiserated together, Jane and I. Both of us have, stretched out behind us now, lives dominated by bladder and vaginal trouble. My cystitis ended after six years but vaginal problems caused by the atrocious over-dosing of antibiotics and absence of self-care or prevention, left years of thrush and a damaged gut where fungus is ever ready to upsurge.

For Jane, who has not been washing properly, cystitis is as rampant now as in her first marriage, but my first point about seeing a good gynaecologist is my uppermost 'instinct' for her. I know full well that vaginal discharges, too, have causes and, since she hasn't had a good gynaecological survey since Luke's birth, I am keen for her to have one.

I gave an extremely firm talk on the bottle washing, with time out on the bathroom demonstration so that, after all these years, we could stop E. Coli bladder infections.

Because Jane was away for August, a date for the gynaecologist was made for early October as convenient to both. During the intervening time Jane's Trimethoprin antibiotics were changed to Tetracycline which calmed down the heavy invasions of E. Coli and reduced the pus in both urine and vaginal specimens.

Follow Up

January 1987, I ran to see what had happened. She had been seen by the gynaecologist I had recommended, who found heavy cervical erosions. Jane had not mentioned these to me in July.

'All the NHS gynaecologists said that there was no need to do anything about them – a lot of women have erosions but they are nothing to worry about.'

'When were they first noticed, do you know?'

'At John's birth, eleven years ago. The obstetrician said he'd seen them, but wouldn't do anything then.'

'Were they still there at Luke's birth?'

'Yes, the professor noted them, but again took no action. I didn't tell you because honestly I thought they meant nothing.'

Well I hit the roof in fury, not at Jane, but at these wretched men who can't do their job properly. If they had an overgrowth of skin cells on the end of their penis, would they want it off? You bet!

Eleven plus years of cervical erosions and eleven plus years of cystitis!

Cervical erosions don't go away. They usually keep growing and they harbour all manner of bacteria. It drips down and contaminates the vulva and urethra. Sexual intercourse breaks the erosion open to spill blood and bacteria into the vagina and cause bladder infection.

The gynaecologist did a pap smear and the lab found it to be Class one normal. Good news. A lot of erosion was cauterized and Jane's next assessment was early February. I mentioned that if erosions are left they grow not only outwards but can also start back into the epidermal layers. Every two months or so reviews should be made and further cautery done until the cervix remains pink and clean all the while.

Jane has still had no sex since 27 May. She is absolutely terrified of getting any more cystitis. There has been no sexually related cystitis but the cautery gave the bacteria already present a chance to raise merry hell and Jane does admit to not bottle washing absolutely faithfully.

I read the riot act about it and gave a pep talk on the erosions and their bearing on the cystitis all these years. Now they were being treated, vaginal health could only improve, *but* if she didn't bottle wash each day after a stool she would keep on re-introducing bowel bacteria on to the perineum.

I also asked that after the February gynaecologist's review, she should, with permission, try gentle sex with dollops of lubricating jelly to pad out an unused vagina and prevent trauma, and also to calm herself. She should have two or three painkillers to relax her a little. We wait and hope.

February – March

Because of deep erosion invasion, the cervix has taken time to heal and the gynaecological review still showed deeper pink patches where healing is progressing slowly. Jane hasn't gathered enough courage for intercourse or even finger penetration and once I heard that all infection has now stopped and bottle washing is at last being done each day, I had to use some strong encouragement and exhortation to get a promise from her that she would try intercourse.

My line ran that unless and until she did try, she would never know what pain-free sex felt like nor would she be ready for intercourse with whatever future husband material ever turned up. Sexual confidence has been badly damaged in this lengthy history of multiple causes for sexual cystitis and I'm damned if I'll give up on her now that so much work and effort has been put in to resolving so many difficulties.

May

The phone rang one evening. Jane announced with some amazement that she and Patrick have started making love and that there has been no cystitis. That she has done this at all is a great relief, not just for her but also for me! I was running out of exhortations! Her mental safeguard is in knowing that a good gynaecologist will always be there to help if she's ever in trouble again, but for the forseeable future all will be well and her battered confidence will return.

Diana Lunges

Diana and her husband Rowan and six-year-old daughter Lizzy came one chilly Sunday afternoon so that Diana could have some counselling. No other time was mutually possible so, whilst Rowan and Lizzy settled downstairs with toys, books, television and hot chocolate, Diana and I had a one hour twenty minute session in my office upstairs.

Diana is tall and elegant both in bearing and dress. At thirty-five years old, she has been married to Rowan for some fifteen years, having met him when she was nine-teen. He is now forty-one and Lizzy, their only child so far, is six years old. Medically referred to me by a urol-ogist, Diana is utterly fed up with her brand of cystitis. All her sexual life she has been in trouble with cystitis but since 1984 the attacks have considerably worsened.

Rowan is a shipping clerk for a cargo line working out of Tilbury Docks. He is largely desk-bound and does not travel. He is a great help in the family unit, supporting Diana and Lizzy and being a co-active spouse. With a great smile he was here supporting Diana fully in her quest for an answer to her misery.

Diana works as a fraud officer investigating false social security claims so she often visits rather unsavoury places. Stress and flexi-time working hours are part of the job, she accepts that. Out of working hours, she is doing an Open University degree course in social science, politics and the changing experiences of women. So here was a mentally gregarious woman, highly motivated and fully occupied, but with a sad sex life and needing my assistance.

Symptoms

Attacks of cystitis. These attacks mostly have a rather unusual feature in that there is no frequency in passing urine at all and no bleeding, though that is not quite so unusual. There is the usual urethral pain and also strong back pain just below the waist on both sides. The area in front of her bladder swells up and she goes in two days, from her normal weight of nine stone two pounds to nine stone seven pounds. After the attack this drops back again. Other sorts of attacks come after intercourse and can start directly with soreness or thirty-six hours later. In 1986 she had about eleven attacks altogether, but none in the three main summer months.

Cystitis has bugged her all her married life, but the non-sexual variety has become stronger and more frequent since Lizzy's third birthday. Since October, and particularly over Christmas, Diana's brand of cystitis has been permanently plugged in!

Lethargy – extreme lethargy – enough to stop her getting to work on time is another symptom and so is thrush because of all the antibiotics given by the doctor for the cystitis. Rowan has thrush also.

Urological Investigations

Mid-stream urine tests	Lots done showing both negative or positive results. The last was January and showed E. Coli.
Intra-venous Pyelogram	One in 1984 which was negative.
Cystoscopy	None.

No other urological work has been undertaken. My next heading is normally gynaecological history but, by chance, Diana mentioned having had an operation for adhesions so I went straight on to general health.

General Health

Appendicitis and removal of the appendix at the age of seventeen. Adhesions began then, and worsened until treated by surgery in 1985 when she was aged thirty-three years. Before the operation, Diana was always constipated but since 1985 has been able to pass a stool each day without straining or the need for laxatives. She has gained weight with the improvement in her digestive system, but as well as cystitis she is worried about the lethargy and tiredness.

Apart from having her tonsils removed when she was a child, Diana has had no other operations.

Gynaecological history

Periods began at the age of eleven, and because they were irregular, heavy and painful, the Pill was recommended when she was seventeen. There was a slight improvement in the cycle regulation but blood loss remained high and there was a full seven-day bleed. At nineteen she met Rowan so the Pill also became a contraceptive. For nine years she remained on the Pill and then had a year's break in 1979. From 1981 to December 1986 the Pill again controlled the difficult cycles and prevented conception. The next period since coming off the Pill is due four days after this counselling.

Children

Lizzy, 1981   A lot of internal and external stitching. Vaginal infection and sporadic removal of afterbirth.

Intercourse

Is sometimes uncomfortable, being dry and producing a sharp pain. This is not always so but when it is there can be an attack of cystitis starting almost immediately. The attack is mostly comprised of urethral pain. The sharp pain during intercourse is situated just inside the vagina and is always in the same place. Not all intercourse has these difficulties and Diana has no 'fear' of it. Even so, the lethargy and other attacks of cystitis are taking their toll on her desire, and it is essential to improve her general condition if we are to give the joy back to her marriage.

Hygiene

Although Diana has read my books, she says that she has not done the bottle washing because her habit each morning is to pass a stool at home and then bath before going to work. Though better than many other routines, this is too haphazard and will account for some of the positive bacterial urine tests. Her bathroom is separate from her lavatory and, whilst there have been discussions about knocking down the inter-connecting wall, it would appear to be technically impossible so this is another reason why she has not felt inclined to bottle wash even though, of course, the problem is easily surmounted as my books show. After intercourse Diana just passes urine but does not bottle wash.

Liquid Intake and Diet

The diet is good, the liquid intake is irregular because of the job. Food is home-cooked and contains minerals, vitamins etc. but the job is so pressured and frenetic that the normal diet does not match the energy output.

Ideas and Suggestions

1 Lethargy can be a symptom of stress, physical debilitation, overwork or any combination of points from any of these general factors.
2 Thrush is coming particularly after the antibiotics. Since Rowan also gets it, both should take a simultaneous course of Nystatin oral tablets.
3 Hormone levels. What are they? A blood test would help in finding out.
4 A good gynaecological examination is needed because it's been three years since the last one.
5 Join in a good health insurance company.
6 Are the childbirth injuries still affecting the part inside the vagina where intercourse sometimes feels painful?
7 Urinary retention on the ninth to the eleventh day of the cycle may be causing the unusual cystitis with the frequency in passing urine. Urinary retention on some days at work is also bad for the bladder.
8 Ovarian hormone activity on the ninth to the eleventh day needs checking.
9 Washing. Bottle wash from now on both after passing a stool and after intercourse. Remember my bathroom demonstration!
10 Some sexual cystitis could be bruising from being tired and dry, some could be infection.
11 Take mineral and vitamin supplements. Buy Ferrograd-C from any pharmacy. It is iron combined with vitamin C and does not make you constipated. The Cantassium Company make all sorts of pure

Vegan tablets for dietary supplement. Look especially for Zinc and Minerals, Magnesium B.13, chromium. Take a four-month course of each, starting with a low dose and going to high then back to a daily maintenance level. It is possible to have a sweat test taken for mineral deficiency.

12 It is extremely important to drink regularly throughout the day and to void regularly (pass urine) as well.

13 Your GP may like to prescribe ten diuretic tablets. Take one each day around the ninth to eleventh day for each of two cycles, just as an experiment to draw off any retaining urine at this time.

14 Use dollops of lubricating jelly before and during intercourse to avoid bruising.

My Comments

Diana is quite obviously overdoing things! A full-time stressful job, a home and family, a degree study course – the mind boggles at it! At thirty-five some of her youthful energy will be declining anyway, but she is helping it no end! Nevertheless, there are other areas of her problems which, if reduced and removed, may lighten the energy drain and let her have a go at finishing off her degree course.

Rowan is being marvellous at home with Lizzy's needs and also very understanding and caring in his attitude to Diana. So the supports that Diana needs for a year or two are there and being made good use of already. How else can I help?

The lethargy in her case stems from a variety of roots:

- Frequent antibiotic therapy, regardless of urine tests.
- Attacks of thrush which can cause real tiredness.
- Heavy bleeding at period time.
- Possible ovulatory and hormonal disturbances.

194

- Insufficient mineral and vitamin intake for energy loss at work.
- Stressful job, stressful cystitis attacks.
- No relaxation 'off duty'.
- Insufficient lovemaking

Inherent in the second, third and fourth points is the monthly cycle. My suggestion of a good gynaecological examination would include hormone work. Assessment, verbal clues and blood testing would put together an accurate idea of what is going on and why certain symptoms of disturbance are occurring. Even whilst on the Pill all those years, there was little, if any, change in the amount of bleeding. That's unusual because most women lose less blood on the Pill. It would be interesting to find out why and whether another hormone combination would reduce the loss. If the loss were reduced, the iron loss and lethargy would be reduced too.

The hormone assessments would also show up ovulatory disturbance, and this point in each monthly cycle is where the major problems show up. Between the ninth and eleventh day, approximately, is the time when an attack of cystitis usually begins.

Diana's brand of cystitis has no frequency, in fact she says, she passes next to no urine at all. She swells up, puts on five pounds in weight, gets awful backache near or in the ovarian region and gets pain in the bladder. This all stops around day twelve.

My suggestion of two cycles using diuretic tablets at this time may well do the trick, but I personally much prefer to go for the root cause in this problem. I feel it is ovarian disturbance that needs sorting out.

During the gynaecological work swabs would be taken and the thrush situation discussed. As well as being caused by courses of antibiotic therapy, thrush can arise from debilitation and from hormone disturbance. A continual watch on prevention is essential, and Rowan should also be treated. The condom is a good safeguard against passing thrush between sexual partners. (See *Victims of Thrush and Cystitis*.)

Whilst the swab-taking or blood-testing is being done, the gynaecologist will know to look very carefully indeed at the current state of the old childbirth scars. Maybe there is a thin one that cannot stand up against the movements in intercourse. Maybe there is a raised flap of scar tissue that needs levelling with cauterization so that it won't affect intercourse. A really expert gynaecologist 'eye' will spot such likely trouble areas that could cause pain in intercourse.

It may be that some cystitis attacks are a whole combination of factors as well as the obviously separate reasons: supposing Diana had a bad day at work – no time to drink, no opportunity to void, intercourse at night without washing afterwards, dry intercourse and on top of all that, she'd forgotten that it was the nine, tenth or eleventh day after the start of the period. Real trouble! For her personally – real trouble!

The hygiene side also had to be worked at seriously because some urine tests are showing E. Coli and other bowel bacteria. I went through the procedure recommended earlier in this book for those women whose lavatories are separate from the other bathroom equipment. Diana, being highly intelligent and motivated to get well will now bottle wash.

Her action plan on leaving counselling is, with my permission and encouragement:

1 Bottle washing after a stool and after intercourse.
2 Mineral and vitamin supplement.
3 Requesting a diuretic from the GP for a two-month trial at ovulation time only.
4 Requesting Nystatin for herself and Rowan.

5 Drinking and voiding more regularly at work.
6 Using dollops of jelly before and during intercourse to stop bruising.
7 Get private health insurance cover.

After two months she will have the insurance plus a good idea of how the diuretic has worked and how helpful the other points have been. This can all then be reported to an expert gynaecologist.

One Year Later

Diana has not got any health insurance nor has she needed a diuretic. Monetarily it became a choice between school fees for Lizzy or health insurance. They chose school fees but sensibly paid out for a private gynaeco-logical check which included a smear. The private specialist found a cervical erosion which was infected and Diana has decided to save up for the operation and steriliz-ation together in the small private hospital near her home.

Diana had left my counselling and, indeed, gone away to do some deep thinking and positive acting. She began by drinking more at work and emptying her bladder at closer intervals. A big regime of recommended mineral and vitamin supplements began and she is still continuing to take them. Most importantly, her job and several related stresses were lessened and unloaded in the autumn. From October the Open University study year ended and in November Diana stopped on-site fraud investigation work. She is involved in office work only. The confront-ational aggression which she met on the doorstep is a thing of the past – a more routine day has eased all the stress.

This is the reason for her periods settling and why she has no need of a diuretic. The cystitis which used to occur from the ninth to the eleventh day hasn't happened for a long while. In fact, since seeing me she has had no thrush and only three attacks of cystitis in one year. None of these took her to the doctor so she has no urine test results. Each of the three attacks went with the self-help management routine and Diana was thrilled at being able to cope by herself.

Rowan has a fully sexually active wife. They make love much more often and Diana has no resulting cystitis. All the tips like the lubricating jelly and bottle washing have made their mark and Diana thanked me for the counselling and the suggestions. It's all down to common sense, self-help and prevention.

Summary

Sexual cystitis even in its mildest, most temporary form is experienced by nearly every woman when starting to have intercourse. 'Honeymoon' bruising escapes very few and if ineffective hygiene allows bacteria to penetrate the bruised, raw skin then a miserable, painful week will ensue.

My main aim in life is to let women know how to avoid such misery. For heaven's sake, show this book to any woman, younger or older, who confides such a problem. To suffer for years, as I did, and many millions more women even longer before my work began, must now become a thing of the past. I lecture to any group and will counsel one-to-one if you really can't sort yourself out from these pages.

I want women to have as much sex as possible. Sex is very good for you and your partner, if you care for the organs used in the proper and appropriate way. If this book is a great help to women then it must also be an eye opener for men, so hand it to yours as well and maybe he'll pick up a few tips. Perhaps he'll even start a discussion on his rating as a lover!

Having lost so much of my own sexuality from my years as a cystitis and thrush victim, I realize that I could have prevented those particular years had I known what I know

now. I am quite determined that you don't suffer like that.

Glossary of Terms

Anaemia   low level of iron in the blood

Anus   opening for passage of faeces

Artery   blood vessel carrying blood *from* the heart

Bacteria   germs

Bicarbonate of soda   baking soda, an alkalizing agent

Bladder   elastic sac in the pelvic region which stores urine

Candida   thrush; a fungus infection of the mouth, vagina and rectum

Catheterization   insertion of a small tube to withdraw urine from the bladder

Cauterization   burning away of infected skin

Cervicitis   any inflammation of the cervix

Cervix   neck of the womb

Colitis   inflammation of the colon (part of the bowel)

Cystoscopy   an operation for investigation of the bladder

Diabetes   illness caused by lack of insulin in the bloodstream

Dialysis   artificial cleansing of the blood by a machine

Dilatation/dilation   enlargement of cervix or urethra by the insertion of rods

Distal urethral stenosis   condition of the bladder during menopause or old age

Diuretic   an agent which stimulates the production of urine

Diverticulitis   inflammation of the bowel

Diverticulum   small false bladder growth

E. Coli   natural bacteria which inhabit the bowel

Enuresis   bed wetting

Episiotomy   an operation on the perineum during difficult childbirth

Epithelium   skin

Foreskin   skin covering the end of the penis

Fungus   growth of detrimental yeast organisms

Gonadotrophin   hormone involved in ovulation

Hexachlorophine   an antiseptic used frequently in hospitals

Hormone   a chemical messenger carrying instructions from glands to organs

Hormone imbalance   incorrect balance of hormones

Hysterectomy   removal of all or part of the internal female sexual organs

IVP   intravenous pyelogram, or kidney X-ray

Labia (majora/minora)   folds of skin which protect urethral and vaginal orifices

Litmus paper   chemical papers able to test for acidity/alkalinity

MSU   mid-stream urine specimen

Menopause   natural process involving termination of menstruation

Micturition   act of passing urine

Micturating cystogram   an X-ray taken during urination

Monilia   thrush; a fungus infection of the mouth, rectum and vagina

Oestrogen   hormone involved in ovulation

Ovulation   release of unfertilized female egg from the ovaries

Perineum   base of the body's trunk containing excretory orifices

Pituitary gland   chief sexual gland of the brain responsible for most hormone activity

Potassium citrate   alkalizing agent

Prostate gland   male sexual gland through which passes the urethra

Pyelitis   kidney disease

Radiographer   specialist in X-ray techniques

Rectum   tube for passing of stools to the outside

Reflux   urine flow in the wrong direction

Renal scarring   scarring of the kidney by constant disease

Sphincter valve   valve attached to the sphincter muscles controlling output of urine

Streptococcus   a form of bacteria

Trichomonas   sexually transmitted disease

Ureters   tubes carrying urine from the kidneys to the bladder

Urethra   tube carrying urine from the bladder

Urethral syndrome   medically unaccountable symptoms of cystitis without bacteria

Urologist   doctor specializing in renal organs

Uterus   womb

Vagina   birth canal

Vaginal thrush   milky, irritative discharge from the vagina

Vaginitis   any inflammation of the vagina

Vein   blood vessel carrying blood *to* the heart

Appendix

List of Carbohydrates

In the ensuing carbohydrate list I have italicised the highest rates.

C = Carbohydrate: P = Protein: F = Fat

Cereals

	Grams	Calories	C	P	F
Arrowroot, uncooked	per 12	61·5	*15*	0	0
Bread, average white	,, 25	74	*15*	3	0
Bread, average brown	,, 25	68	*15*	1·5	0
Corn Flakes	,, 12	45	10	1	0
Macaroni, boiled	,, 50	58·5	10	2	1
Oatmeal, raw	,, 12	68	10	2	2
Rice, uncooked	,, 12	51	12·5	0	0
Sago, uncooked	,, 12	51	12·5	0	0

Sugary Foods

	Grams	Calories	C	P	F
Chocolate, average, milk	per 12	84	7·5	1	5
Chocolate, average, plain	,, 12	62	7·5	1	3
Golden syrup, as purchased	,, 12	51	12·5	0	0
Honey, as purchased	,, 12	51	12·5	0	0
Jam, average	,, 7	20·5	5	0	0
Marmalade, ordinary	,, 12	51	12·5	0	0
Marmalade, sugarless, reliable make		Negligible			
Sugar, one large lump	,, 12	20·5	5	0	0

Milk

	Grams	Calories	C	P	F
Buttermilk	per 87	42	5	3	1
Milk, fresh	,, { 25	19	1·5	1	1
	,, { 87	67	5	3·5	3·5
Milk, skimmed	,, 87	41·5	5	4	0·5
Milk, condensed, unsweetened	,, 25	61	5	3	3
Milk, dried	,, 12	67	5	3·5	3·5

Fruit and Nuts

	Grams	Calories	C	P	F
Apple, with skin	per 50	20·5	5	0	0
Apricots, fresh, with stones	,, 75	25	5	1	0
Banana, average size	,, 75	61·5	15	0	0
Figs, green, raw	,, 50	26	5	1	0
Grapefruit, with skin	,, 175	22	5	0·5	0
Grapes, fresh	,, 25	20	5	0	0
Melon, edible part	,, 87	23	5	1	0
Nuts, almond	,, 12	78	0·5	3	7
Nuts, brazil	,, 12	86	0·5	2	8
Nuts, chestnut	,, 12	68	5	3	4
Nuts, walnut	,, 12	74	0·5	2	7
Olives	,, 25	46·5	0	0	5
Peaches, fresh, with stones	,, 56	22·5	5	0·5	0
Pears, fresh, with skin	,, 75	27	6	0·5	0
Pineapple, fresh, edible part	,, 37	20·5	5	0	0
Plums, ripe, Victoria (with stones)	,, 50	20·5	5	0	0
Rhubarb		Negligible			

Dairy Products

	Grams	Calories	C	P	F
Cheese	per 12	50–70 varies roughly			
Eggs, one average whole egg	,, –	76	–	6	5·5

Fish

	Grams	Calories	C	P	F
Cod, boiled	per 75	61	0	15	0
Crab, edible part	,, 50	58	0	10	2
Haddock, boiled	,, 75	82	0	20	0
Halibut, boiled	,, 37	58	0	10	2
Herring, fresh	,, 50	112	0	10	8
Kipper, boiled	,, 37	76	0	10	4
Mackerel, boiled	,, 75	114	0	15	6
Plaice, steamed	,, 50	50	0	10	1
Salmon, boiled	,, 75	142	0	15	9
Skate, boiled	,, 50	50	0	10	1
Turbot, cooked	,, 75	60	0	15	0
Whiting, steamed	,, 50	41	0	10	0

Meat

	Grams	Calories	C	P	F
Bacon, fat, fried	per 25	160	0	5	15
Bacon, lean	,, 37	220	0	10	20
Beef, average roast	,, 50	201	0	15	15
Beef, roast lean	,, 50	87	0	15	3
Ham, boiled, lean only	,, 37.5	94	0	10	6
Kidneys, cooked	,, 50	87	0	25	3
Lamb, roast	,, 75	175	0	20	10
Liver, cooked	,, 50	141	0	15	9
Mutton, roast	,, 50	168	0	15	12
Mutton chop, lean, grilled	,, 50	224	0	20	16
Pork, roast	,, 50	229	0	15	18
Rabbit, stewed	,, 50	89	0	15	3
Sweetbreads, cooked	,, 37	78	0	10	4
Tongue, ox, tinned	,, 37	162	0	10	13
Veal, roast	,, 50	156	0	20	8

Poultry and Game

	Grams	Calories	C	P	F
Chicken, roast or boiled	per 50	103	0	15	4·5
Duck, roast	,, 37	134	0	10	10
Goose, roast	,, 50	173	0	15	12
Turkey, roast	,, 50	89	0	15	3

Vegetables

	Grams	Calories	C	P	F
Asparagus, fresh, boiled (edible part)	per 225	16	2·5	7·5	0
Beans, broad	,, 62	33	5	3	0
Beans, butter	,, 50	56	10	4	0
Beans, haricot	,, 50	56	10	4	0
Beans, French	,, 225	16	2·5	1·5	0
Beans, scarlet runner		Negligible			
Beetroot, boiled once	,, 33	25	5	1	0
Brussels sprouts					
Cabbage, spring		May be considered negligible			
Cabbage, winter					
Carrots, boiled once	,, 100	23	5	0·5	0
Cauliflower					
Celery, raw		May be considered negligible			
Celery, baked					
Cress					
Cucumber, raw, without skin	,, 150	14	2·5	1	0
Cucumber, boiled	,, 175	11	2·5	0	0
Lettuce raw		Negligible			
Mushrooms		Negligible			
Onions, boiled once	,, 87	14	2·5	0·5	0
Peas, boiled once, green fresh	,, 50	70	14	2	0·5
Peas, tinned, green	,, 50	57	10	4	0
Peas, green, dried	,, 50	57	10	4	0
Potatoes, raw or boiled once	,, 25	22·5	5	0·5	0
Spinach, boiled once	,, 175	46	2·5	9	0
Tomatoes, raw, cooked or tinned	,, 100	20	3	1	0
Watercress, raw	,, 25	Negligible			

This list has been reproduced by kind permission of the Hamlyn Publishing Group.

Bibliography and Further Reading

Brudenell, J. M., and Peel, J. H., *Textbook of Gynaecology*, (Heinemann Medical Books, 1943).

Cleave, T. L., *The Saccharine Disease*, (John Wright and Sons, 1966).

Cooper, Wendy, *No Change*, new ed., (Arrow Books, 1988).

Dechesne, B., Pons, C., Schellen, A., *Sexuality and Handicap*, (Woodhead-Faulkner, 1985).

Delvin, David, *The Book of Love*, (New English Library, 1974).

Fairburn, C. G., *Sexual Problems and Their Management*, (Churchill Livingstone Medical Text, Longman Group, 1983).

Mendelsohn, Robert S., MD, *Male Practice*, (Chicago: Contemporary Books, 1981).

Ritter, Henry, MD, *From Man to Man*, (New York: Harper and Row, 1979).

Shanson, D. C., *Microbiology in Clinical Practice*, (John Wright and Sons, 1982).

Stewart, W. F. R., *The Sexual Side of Handicap*, (Woodhead-Faulkner, 1979).

Wingate, Peter, *Penguin Medical Encyclopedia*, (Penguin Reference Books, 1972).